HOMOEOPATHY FOR EVERYONE

Sheila Gibson qualified in medicine at Glasgow University in 1962, having previously acquired an honours B.Sc. degree in biochemistry. Her interests have always been in the field of research, first in toxicology and then in genetics. Since joining the staff of the Glasgow Homoeopathic Hospital, where she is currently research co-ordinator in the Department of Creative Therapeutics, she has been active in research in allergy, rheumatology, multiple sclerosis and the post-viral syndrome. The role of diet and nutrition in disease production and health maintenance has been a major interest along with an appreciation of many aspects of the alternative health scene, their spheres of action and their inter-relationships.

Robin Gibson was educated in Edinburgh. After qualifying in dentistry from Edinburgh University, he studied medicine in Glasgow where he qualified in 1960. While still a student, he encountered homoeopathy, and after specializing in paediatrics his interest was stimulated by his successful use of homoeopathic remedies in the treatment of croup in young children. He studied homoeopathy in Glasgow and London. Since becoming a consultant physician at the Glasgow Homoeopathic Hospital, he has exercised his research interests in the fields of nutrition, posture, allergy, rheumatology and, more recently, multiple sclerosis, investigating the potential of a number of disciplines and techniques complementary to homoeopathy. His trials in rheumatology were the first homoeopathic clinical trials to be published in an orthodox medical journal. At present he is head of the Department of Creative Therapeutics at the Glasgow Homoeopathic Hospital and is pioneering new methods of disease management linked with researchers in London and America.

SHEILA AND ROBIN GIBSON

HOMOEOPATHY FOR EVERYONE

ARKANA

ARKANA

Published by the Penguin Group
Penguin Books Ltd, 27 Wrights Lane, London W8 5TZ, England
Viking Penguin, a division of Penguin Books USA Inc.
375 Hudson Street, New York, New York 10014, USA
Penguin Books Australia Ltd, Ringwood, Victoria, Australia
Penguin Books Canada Ltd, 2801 John Street, Markham, Ontario, Canada L3R 1B4
Penguin Book (NZ) Ltd, 182–190 Wairau Road, Auckland 10, New Zealand

Penguin Books Ltd, Registered Offices: Harmondsworth, Middlesex, England

Published in Penguin Books 1987
Published by Arkana 1991
10 9 8 7 6 5 4 3 2

Printed in England by Clays Ltd, St Ives plc
Typeset in 11/13 Monophoto Plantin

We wish to dedicate this book
to the future of homoeopathy

There is a principle which is a bar against all information, which is proof against all arguments and which cannot fail to keep a man in everlasting ignorance – that principle is contempt prior to investigation

Herbert Spencer, 1820–1903

CONTENTS

LIST OF FIGURES

ACKNOWLEDGEMENTS

We wish to thank all our colleagues and patients for their help and support, and in particular, Dr Gordon Flint, Dr Anton van Rhijn, Dr Andreas Pfretschner, Mr Jim Crawford of Nelsons, the late Mr P. J. Thomas, who was our librarian, Miss Margaret Cooper of the Hahnemann Society, and Mrs Nan Donaldson and Miss Isobel Smith, our long-suffering neighbours.

CHAPTER ONE

HOMOEOPATHY

IN ACTION

A young man of seventeen was admitted to an infectious diseases unit because he was coughing up blood, had bleeding gums and had not felt well for two to three years. Tuberculosis was suspected, but X-rays and blood tests proved negative. Despite intensive investigation no diagnosis was made but, in the course of routine examination, he was found to have an enlarged spleen which extended for about one hand's breadth below the rib cage. No other abnormality was found and he was discharged from the hospital after six weeks.

However he continued to feel unwell and he was fully investigated in the haematology unit of a large teaching hospital. Again the only abnormality found was the large spleen. This was not considered to be particularly harmful, as his blood count was within normal limits, and there was no evidence of increased breakdown of his red blood cells. One of the functions of the spleen is to act as a reservoir for blood cells and to remove and destroy damaged red cells. The spleen was therefore not removed. No therapy was given, but he was reviewed at six-monthly intervals. He continued his work as a printer but never really felt well. He himself attributed most of his symptoms to his enlarged spleen, despite the reassurance of the consultant that this was not the case. The opinion of the haematology unit was that this feeling of debility was the result of knowing that he had an enlarged spleen and that it was 'all in the mind'.

At the age of thirty-two he attended the homoeopathic

out-patient clinic. Despite his by now thick case-sheet – as he was still being reviewed every six months – there had been no change in the size of his spleen or in his general symptoms over the previous fifteen years. His gums also continued to bleed sporadically. A careful homoeopathic history was taken and *Ceanothus americanus*,[1] a blue-flowered shrub used by Compton Burnett for the treatment of spleen conditions, was considered to be the most appropriate remedy. The drug picture of ceanothus – that is, the totality of the symptoms – includes that of a low-spirited patient who is fearful that he or she will become unfit for work. There is a feeling of general debility which makes work difficult and a burden, right-sided headache, discomfort in the region of the spleen, ulceration of the mouth, poor appetite and a constant feeling of being cold. There is also a restricted feeling in the chest, palpitations and generalized weakness. This patient was therefore given a dose of ceanothus.

When he was reviewed two weeks later, the spleen surprisingly was scarcely palpable. The patient himself had much more energy and no longer felt the need to take alcohol in an attempt to lessen his sense of ill-being. After a further two weeks, no spleen was detected and the patient felt better than he had since he was a young man. Within six months of his first visit to the homoeopathic clinic, he had set up his own printing business which he ran successfully over the five-year follow-up.

He was seen at regular intervals over this period. He found that every eighteen months or so he would have a flu-like illness and on examination the tip of the spleen could be felt once more. A further dose of ceanothus rapidly restored his sense of well-being and the spleen also regressed. Eventually he purchased a bottle of the remedy so that he could take it when required without having to come to the clinic.

A thirty-year-old patient had marked swelling of the hands and feet, accompanied by pain, stiffness and inability to close his hands satisfactorily. He had had these symptoms for several months and had recently been diagnosed as suffering from rheumatoid arthritis. He was invited to take part in a trial of homoeopathy which we were carrying out. It was explained to him that the trial would last for six months, and that during the first three months he might either have the active therapy or the placebo (the inactive therapy), but that during the second three months he would be given the active remedy. The purpose of the trial was to assess the efficacy of homoeopathy compared with placebo in rheumatoid arthritis. The protocol was such that during the first three months of the trial neither the prescribing doctors nor the patients knew who was receiving the active therapy. In order to give all the patients the chance of receiving the active therapy, during the second three months of the trial all had homoeopathy but again neither the prescribing doctors nor the patients knew who had changed therapies until the code was broken at the end of the six-month period of the trial.

Apart from his pain, stiffness and swelling, this patient's outstanding characteristics were a marked fear of heights, an aversion to fat, a tendency to sleep on his abdomen and a tendency to faint in stuffy rooms. He was upset by pork and could not tolerate hot drinks. These characteristics pointed to pulsatilla, the Pasque flower, as being the most appropriate remedy. This was duly prescribed and he was given one dose a month. For the first three months there was no improvement at all, but within two days of his fourth powder – that is, the beginning of the fourth month – he showed a dramatic response and the swelling, pain and stiffness completely disappeared. On breaking the code at the completion of the trial, it was discovered that he had been on the placebo for the first three months, but responded dramatically as soon as he received the active treatment, the pulsatilla.

He has now been followed up for eight years. He has needed the occasional dose of pulsatilla when there has been a slight return of joint pain and swelling. He remains very well and has long ago discontinued the orthodox anti-inflammatory drugs which he was taking when he entered the double-blind trial.

In both these cases the complaints were primarily physical, but homoeopathic remedies are equally effective for mental-emotional problems. This is illustrated by the interesting case of a woman of sixty-four who was admitted to the homoeopathic hospital with a bad attack of lobar pneumonia. Although she was improving slowly in the ward, she was a very difficult patient. The nurses found her almost impossible to manage, as she was extremely restless and unsettled, and was always trying to leave the hospital. She wanted to get home and assured the staff that she had someone who would stay with her and look after her. However her son, a doctor, telephoned to say that this was not true and commented that she became very anxious in an enclosed space and had to get out for long walks, even when she was at home. She became desperately unhappy when restricted.

These comments suggested the remedy *Argentum nitricum*. Patients requiring this remedy often suffer from considerable anxiety and apprehension, particularly in enclosed spaces. It was therefore given to her and within two hours she was a totally changed person: quiet and relaxed and no longer disturbing the ward. The nurses and doctors were amazed at the transformation. Thereafter she was quite happy to remain in the hospital until her pneumonia had cleared up.

The power of homoeopathic remedies to influence moods and attitudes is again well illustrated by the following bizarre case which concerns a woman of about thirty-four years of age. A cardiac surgeon gave a lecture at a clinical symposium on a case which involved a boy of about five years old – an only child whose father had been working in Jamaica – who developed a flu-like illness. As he did not respond to the treatment given there, he was flown home and admitted to a top paediatric unit. Extensive investigations were carried out and he was diagnosed as having an infectious cardiomyopathy (infection of the heart muscle). The main clinical finding was an enlarged heart. However, despite what seemed to be the appropriate therapy, he continued to deteriorate and the heart continued to enlarge. The only investigation which had not been done was cardiac catheterization as this was considered too risky in an infected heart. However, as deterioration continued and there was no response to therapy after several months, this procedure was finally carried out eight months after his original admission to hospital. Much to the paediatricians' surprise, it was discovered that the boy's heart was normal in size and that what had been thought to be a large heart was a large heart tumour which was pushing the heart out of place and producing the symptoms of heart failure which he was experiencing. At this point the cardiac surgeon was called in and asked to operate on what was, by now, an extremely ill child. The operation was successful but the child, unfortunately, was so debilitated that he had a very stormy post-operative period and finally died some weeks later in spite of everything which could be done for him.

The tragic thing about the case was that this type of tumour is eminently operable; it is one of the few tumours which, if once removed, does not tend to recur, and the child should have had a reasonable life expectancy. The mother, understandably, was very upset, and felt that she could never forgive the paediatricians for causing, as she saw it, the death of her child. The fact that he was an only child, and that she had been told that she could never have any more children, made the situation even more tragic. A friendship developed between the parents and the surgeon which in some way mitigated the mother's distress as she felt that she still had a link with her lost son.

About a year after this lecture, a couple appeared at the homoeopathic out-patient department. The wife was in a terrible state of anguish and almost incoherent with grief. It turned out that they were the parents of the child who had been the subject of the surgeon's lecture. The surgeon himself had died unexpectedly just a few weeks previously and the parents felt that they had lost their last link with their child. The mother particularly felt that she could never forgive the paediatric unit for having failed to diagnose her son in time, although the error, in the context of the medical history, was understandable.

The most appropriate remedy for this state of mind was staphisagria (a remedy for suppressed or harboured resentment) and this was given to the mother. It was explained to her that her feelings were wholly understandable but that she was holding herself prisoner in a time capsule which was helping no one, least of all herself. No attempt was made to give any psychotherapy.

When reviewed two weeks later, she was a totally different person. Her whole outlook was much more positive and she had decided to take up a job as a librarian, whereas previously she had just been moping about the house. Several weeks later she was able to forgive the paediatricians and to free herself totally from the negative situation in which she had been trapped. She is now living a happy, normal life and hoping, perhaps over-optimistically, to have another child.

The amazing ability of staphisagria to influence deep levels of the psyche is further illustrated by the case of a woman who came to the homoeopathic clinic when she was forty-three. Her story was that seventeen years previously, when she was nursing her third child, she discovered that her husband, who had never to her knowledge been unfaithful before, was going out with another woman. Understandably, she was deeply wounded and resentful. There she was, tied at home with another baby, while *he* was gallivanting around with someone else. Her husband quickly dropped his new girlfriend, bought his wife flowers and became a model husband. Nevertheless, although she wanted to forgive him, she found that she could not. Her body also could not forgive him. Her endocrine (hormone) system had obviously been so deeply disturbed that she proceeded to have persistent menstrual bleeding, which caused her a great deal of inconvenience and effectively put an end to their marital relationship.

Extensive investigations by many gynaecologists revealed no obvious cause for the disturbance and no treatment had any effect. This went on for seventeen years, until she came to the homoeopathic clinic. She was, by this time, quite desperate. In view of the history, staphisagria was given. When seen three weeks later, she commented happily that she had had a normal period for the first time since the birth of her last child. She had a second dose of staphisagria two weeks later and when reviewed in a further two months was feeling very well, better than she had done for years. She also commented that at long last she had been able to forgive her husband.

Frights also can have a remarkably deep and long-lasting effect on health and well-being. A woman of about thirty was competent and well-organized. One night her husband had to be rushed to hospital as a sudden emergency with a bleeding duodenal ulcer, and required over twenty pints of blood. The situation was extremely frightening for her; she was very shocked and afraid that he would die. However, after an emergency operation, he made a successful recovery and life apparently returned to normal.

Nonetheless, some months later she became anxious and fearful. She developed agoraphobia which made it impossible for her to go out on her own, episodes of tachycardia (racing heart), panic states and bouts of acute anxiety and fear. She did not respond to any conventional medication nor to psychotherapy.

Some two years later she attended the homoeopathic clinic with her husband. Because of the history of fright there was a choice of remedies: opium or aconite. She was given opium, but three weeks later there was still no improvement. She was then given aconite, and within a day felt much better and lost all her previous fears and anxieties. She rapidly returned to normal and has now been followed up for over three years, remaining very well and requiring no further treatment.

A little boy of four was on holiday with his parents at a coastal caravan site when he slipped and fell into a cess-pit. Although he was very quickly rescued and appeared to be unharmed physically, this horrifying experience had a profound effect on him. He became completely withdrawn, would not play or speak to anyone and did not want to eat. All he would do was sit tucked into a dark corner, apparently totally shocked. He was brought to the clinic about a week after the incident – a pathetic, listless, withdrawn child who had responded to no treatment so far given. He was prescribed a dose of opium and by the following day he was smiling and talking and had recovered his previously good appetite.

Not only mental-emotional problems but cases of apparently obvious tissue damage can sometimes respond remarkably well to homoeopathic treatment. This is illustrated by the case of a young man who in 1971 developed weakness of the muscles of the face and difficulties in focusing his eyes. In 1972 a consultant neurologist diagnosed him as a case of myasthenia gravis, a disorder of the system which transfers nerve impulses from the nerves to the muscles. At that time the treatment for patients with myasthenia who were continuing to deteriorate was to remove the thymus gland, which is one of the major centres of antibody production. It had been found that removal of the thymus could produce an improvement in a proportion of the cases treated. Accordingly, the patient had his thymus removed in June 1972 with no obvious improvement but after the operation he suffered from severe weakness for three months.

When seen at the homoeopathic clinic in March 1974 he was still very weak and was taking the orthodox treatment for myasthenia gravis: six neostigmine tablets a day together with some atropine which acts as an antidote for some of the side-effects of neostigmine. He did not feel at all well and was seeking an alternative treatment to the drugs which gave him diarrhoea, though this could be controlled by taking other drugs.

A history was taken which revealed that as a child he had been a sleep-walker. He sweated excessively on his feet, hands, arms and head. This was so bad that on occasion he had to change his socks twice a day and his shirt, and often also his jacket, once a day. He was better when warm, worse when cold, and got achy in damp weather. He liked cold foods and drinks rather than hot ones, slept badly and often lay awake worrying about his work. This combination of symptoms, especially the somnambulism and the excessive sweating, suggested the remedy silica, which has the general picture of a patient who is pale and feeble and has marked sweating of the hands and feet. There is a lack of strength and confidence and a dread of failure, and often a history of sleep-walking. Such patients often prefer cold foods and drinks as hot foods make them perspire. Milk often upsets them. They often sleep badly and lie awake worrying. He was given a dose of silica.

When he was seen again one month later, he had reduced his orthodox medication to five neostigmine tablets a day and had lost six pounds in weight – no doubt due to his increased activity. The sweating of the feet had improved and he could now, if wished, go for two days without changing his socks. He was sleeping better and was much more self-assured.

No further treatment was given at this stage and when he was seen again six weeks later, he was feeling much better. He was now taking two neostigmine and no atropine tablets a day and had no diarrhoea. The silica was now repeated. Two months later he was even better than at the previous visit and this improvement held after another month. However, he still needed two neostigmine tablets a day. At this point he was given a higher potency of silica and two months later reported that he had been off the neostigmine for five weeks and had no sweating of the feet. He was given a further high dose of silica and three and a half months later reported that he had required only six neostigmine tablets since last being seen. He has been followed up over the past ten years. Currently he is holding down a very responsible job and has a handicap of three at golf. In this time he has required only two further repeats of silica and no other medication.

Though natural remissions can occur in myasthenia gravis, they are usually short-lasting and normally occur in the early stages of the disease. In the case of this patient, the marked improvement in all his symptoms – for example, his sweating and his sleep pattern, as well as his weakness – suggest that his remission was due to the remedy which he had been given. Had the remission been spontaneous the sweating, sleep pattern and self-image would not have improved as well.

Homoeopathy is also eminently successful in the treatment of allergy. In this case, the remedy is prepared from the substance to which the patient is sensitive or allergic. The use of such remedies is not homoeopathy in the strictly classical sense and has been given the name isopathy. Isopathy is the use of an antigen (the sensitizing agent in allergy) in homoeopathically potentized form to treat cases of allergy or hypersensitivity to that particular material. A number of standard allergy remedies now exist in the materia medica (the list of remedies); the ones used most frequently probably being house dust 200 for the treatment of house-dust-mite allergy and the hay fever remedies which include mixed-grass pollens, ambrosia, ragweed, timothy grass and beach grass. Remedies also exist prepared from cat and dog hair and horse dander, as well as from a number of moulds.

House-dust-mite allergy is probably the most prevalent allergy in this country today. Although the classic picture is that of a child with asthma and eczema, a common presentation is the child who develops a slight rash in the first few months of life and goes on to develop recurrent sore throats and coughs which become more noticeable when the child is moved from cot to bed. The reason for this is that a cot usually has a plastic-covered mattress whereas a bed does not. The house-dust mite lives in the mattress, feeding on skin scales which have been broken down by fungi and moulds. Any new upholstered mattress is reckoned to be heavily infested with house-dust mites within three months. Other symptoms of allergy to this mite include enlarged tonsils and adenoids, recurrent abdominal pain – with or without vomiting – general tiredness, irritability, muscle pains, perennial rhinitis (constantly stuffed or runny nose), catarrh and ulceration of the mouth.

The efficacy of a homoeopathic preparation of house dust and the wide spectrum of symptoms which it can alleviate are illustrated by the following cases:

The first is that of a little girl of four who had had severe asthma for two years and had been treated with a variety of inhalers with very little effect. When she was seen at the homoeopathic out-patient clinic, skin-testing showed that she was strongly allergic to house-dust mite. Her mother was advised to buy her a solid foam, plastic-covered mattress, a washable Terylene pillow and bedding which could be washed frequently. The base of the bed was to be simple springs or wooden slats. All bedding had to be washed every two to three months to prevent a build-up of the mite. A solid foam, plastic-covered mattress prevents penetration of the mattress by the mite. The child was also given one dose of homoeopathically prepared house dust. Following this treatment of both the child and her bed the asthma cleared up, and she was able to discontinue all other medication. She was followed up for the next five years and kept very well, but required a dose of house dust two to three times a year.

Another case is that of a girl who was a singer in a night-club. She attended the clinic with loss of voice which had prevented her from singing for two years. It was found that she had slight bronchospasm (wheeze) and skin-testing showed that she was very sensitive to the house-dust mite. She was advised on how to treat her bed and given a dose of homoeopathically prepared house dust. Following this she rapidly recovered her voice and was able to resume her singing in the night-club. However, after she had been back at work for about a month, her symptoms gradually returned. Inquiry revealed no problems with the bed, which is usually the main source of exposure to the house-dust mite. As most people do, however, she was hanging up her clothes – including the cabaret garments which she wore in the night-club – in her bedroom. She was advised to change her cabaret outfit whenever she came in from work and to hang it up in the hall. When she did this, she had no further symptoms. It was felt that in the crowded, enclosed atmosphere of the night-club her clothes were picking up sufficient house-dust mites to affect her.

A girl of about seven had episodes of cyclical vomiting, often on a Monday morning, and was regularly absent from school on account of this. When she was admitted to a children's hospital the vomiting improved, and it was thought that it was psychological in origin and that the mother was being over-protective. There was a family history of allergy and skin-testing showed that the child was strongly sensitized to house-dust mite. When this was treated with the usual advice about the bed and a dose of the homoeopathic preparation of house dust, the problem completely cleared up. The child felt very much better and was no longer absent from school. The mother also was much relieved as she did not believe that she was being over-protective and was delighted to find that there was a physical reason for her daughter's problem.

A number of children with night cough and recurrent episodes of unexplained high temperature were found to be house-dust-mite allergic. When this was treated, there were no further episodes of high temperature, the coughs cleared up and there was a marked improvement in well-being. It was also found that a number of children who apparently had stress-induced asthma no longer developed asthma, even when stressed, once the main cause of the problem – the house-dust-mite allergy – was treated. A few cases of unexplained fainting on sudden exertion were also found to be linked to house-dust allergy and improved with the usual management.

Other presentations of house-dust-mite allergy include general tiredness with no other symptoms and unexplained, persistent itch of the eyelids, particularly in older patients. A few cases of severe, intermittent, unexplained abdominal colic in adults, lasting for two to three days, and occurring every six weeks or so for no obvious reason, have also been found to be manifestations of house-dust-mite allergy, and improved when this was treated.

A dramatic case of house-dust-mite allergy was a man in his mid-thirties who attended the out-patient clinic with a nine-year history of a recurrent cycle of illness which started with a herpetic eruption (cold sore) on both lips. This was followed by the appearance of ulcers in his mouth and then a skin rash on the backs of his hands which gradually became very tender over a period of about four weeks. These problems were accompanied by a feeling of lethargy and exhaustion. After this time all the symptoms gradually improved, only to recur two weeks later. The whole cycle was repeated roughly every six weeks.

On questioning it was found that he had had slight bronchospasm at the age of eighteen, and skin-testing showed that he was strongly sensitized to house-dust mite. He was advised on how to treat his bed (in those days a simple polythene cover for the mattress was suggested) and given a homoeopathic preparation of house dust. His condition rapidly cleared up.

About a year later, he decided to change the plastic cover on his mattress and the following day he was admitted to hospital with a terrible rash on his face, hands and arms – the areas which had been exposed to the mites – and a temperature of 104°F. He was severely ill and had been admitted to hospital as a case of encephalitis (inflammation of the brain), but a lumbar puncture failed to show any infection and he was discharged home. He was admitted to our own unit where he responded quickly to the homoeopathic preparation of house dust, though the rash on his hands and face took six weeks to clear up. He was advised to buy a new mattress and to cover it completely with a good quality polyvinyl cover before using it, so that he would never again be at risk of a similar exposure. He has remained well since.

If the remedy for a particular allergy does not exist in the materia medica, it can be made simply enough if one knows what the allergen is. A nineteen-year-old laboratory technician developed an allergy to chloroform which caused severe flaking of the skin of his hands. This was very awkward because his work entailed lead estimations which, in those days, were carried out by coupling the lead with a substance called dithizone in a chloroform solution. He was therefore handling a great deal of chloroform in the course of his daily work. He was sent along to the homoeopathic clinic with a sample of the chloroform and a potency was prepared from this and given to him. His hands cleared up within a day or two and although he continued to handle the chloroform regularly he had no further trouble.

A patient of thirty-four was admitted to hospital with unexplained breathlessness which had been present for about two years. It improved while he was in the unit and no cause was found. However, as soon as he returned home, the breathlessness reappeared and he had to walk very slowly, like an old man, on account of it. On further questioning, it turned out that there was a chemical works near his home which emitted much formaldehyde vapour. He was given the appropriate remedy – a potency of formalin which markedly improved his symptoms. He kept a number of powders to take should the symptoms recur.

A similar case involved a girl who had a corneal transplant. Before she had this operation, she enjoyed the odd glass of wine with no after-effects. After the operation, however, she discovered that if she drank wine the area of the transplant became very itchy – to such an extent that she was forced to forgo wine altogether. A homoeopathic preparation of wine was made and administered to her after which she had no further trouble.

The effects of homoeopathy are not confined to humans. Animals can respond too, sometimes in surprising ways.

We once had a rabbit who developed a swollen, discharging left eye. She also became very quiet, subdued and lethargic, quite unlike her previously frisky self. Silica seemed indicated as the most appropriate remedy, but treatment with various potencies had no effect. A short time afterwards we were visited by a colleague who also thought that silica was the correct remedy. When told that it had already been tried, he suggested giving it in a really high or strong potency. This was done and the following morning we were greeted by an alert and frisky rabbit whose eye was very much better. But these were not the only results. Silica is a remedy which is often needed by cats. Our rabbit suddenly developed a taste for bacon rinds, cold meat, fish and cheese – most unrabbitlike items of diet. She continued to enjoy her normal rabbit-type foods, but also developed a taste for the kinds of food that cats like. She kept these tastes and preferences for the rest of her life.

A colleague's dog was hit by a car – an accident which gave it a considerable fright but did not cause a fracture, although there was considerable bruising. The dog was given the appropriate injury remedies by his owner but in spite of this the animal continued to drag his hind legs. This went on for a number of months without any improvement. The history was reviewed, and because of the fright it was reckoned that the dog must have experienced at the time of the accident, opium was suggested. This remedy soon put things to rights and had the dog prancing around again, as well as ever.

The cases described in this chapter are just a few of the many that could be quoted to illustrate the wide variety of problems that can be treated successfully with homoeopathy. The results of such treatment can be far-reaching and sometimes dramatic but this is not to say that homoeopathy can help every patient or every type of illness. It is of particular value in injuries and accidents, both for the physical damage sustained and for the fright or shock which often accompanies it; in acute infections such as colds, sore throats, acute fevers, influenza and the acute infectious diseases like measles, whooping cough or chicken-pox; in allergies and hypersensitivity reactions of all types, whether to natural substances such as house-dust mite, grass pollens, iodine or nickel, or a host of man-made and other chemical agents like formalin or chloroform; and in emotional upsets, bereavements and other grief states, resentments, menstrual irregularities and sexual problems. In conditions such as these the effect of homoeopathic treatment can be rapid and can often avoid the need for antibiotics or other conventional therapies, but it can where necessary be used in conjunction with orthodox treatments as it works in a different way, strengthening and speeding up the healing response of the body.

Homoeopathy, however, is equally effective in many chronic conditions such as heart, chest, stomach, intestinal, bladder and other genito-urinary problems, arthritis and rheumatism of various types, skin complaints such as eczema, psoriasis and dermatitis, migraines and other chronic headaches, some neurological disorders, psychosomatic diseases and anxiety states. Some cases of cancer, too, will respond to homoeopathic treatment, particularly if the therapist succeeds in selecting the correct remedy. Again homoeopathic and conventional therapies can be used together if necessary.

Homoeopathy's success in treating emotional and psychological problems may be the reason why it is often considered to be merely a placebo therapy or some form of psychotherapy or suggestion. However, as we shall see in Chapter 4, the physical and psychological or emotional-mental aspects of an individual are intimately interlinked, and factors affecting one invariably affect the others as well. It is, therefore, inherently unlikely that one aspect can be treated without having an effect, however small, on the others. The fact that one can feel under par emotionally if one has a physical pain, and experience a lift of the spirits if this is suddenly relieved, illustrates the operation of this interdependence even at the most superficial of levels.

Homoeopathy has always recognized the relationship between the physical and psychological aspects of an illness, and all the deep-acting remedies have physical, emotional and mental symptoms in their drug pictures. What these are and how they were derived will be described later on.

Homoeopathy's ability, then, to improve the psychological state of the patient does not mean that the treatment itself is just placebo or 'all in the mind'. This would imply that only patients who were open to such suggestion, or had faith in the treatment, would be able to respond to it. However, animals, babies and young children, who have no idea what they are being treated with, respond just as well as – and in many cases even better than – adults in whom the suggestion of a placebo effect could be valid in some cases.

It is, therefore, highly unlikely that the clinical improvements obtained using homoeopathy are merely a placebo effect. We are left with the inescapable fact that homoeopathy does work, that the results obtained using it are real and valid. In later chapters we shall go into some of the theories as to how the remedies may exert their effects and into some of the evidence to support the claim that they do.

CHAPTER TWO

A VISIT TO

A HOMOEOPATHIC

DOCTOR

There is a popular notion abroad that homoeopathy is effective only because the doctor spends a long time talking to the patient and this is thought to be the main therapy involved. Some patients may be a little apprehensive of consulting a homoeopathic doctor, not knowing what to expect. They may have heard that such a doctor asks many strange and inconsequential questions that have little relevance they can see to their problems.

There is, however, a good reason why a homoeopathic doctor likes to spend longer with patients than possibly the average orthodox practitioner does. It is necessary if he is to elicit from the patient all the information about symptoms and signs which is required to match the problem with an appropriate remedy. As it were, an identikit of the patient and his illness which matches the features of one of the many remedies available to homoeopathic doctors has to be built up. The interview will begin along similar lines to that conducted by a conventional doctor with inquiry as to what is troubling the patient, how long the condition has been present, any past history of other or similar complaints and a full family history.

The homoeopathic doctor, however, must enlarge on the information normally obtained, since it is the patient in all his or her aspects, and not just the presenting problem, which is being treated. The doctor will inquire about how

the condition began and particularly about any precipitating causes there may have been, such as an injury,
being ch.'lled, an infection, bereavement, fright, anxiety or
deep-seated, smouldering resentment. This is important
because the remedy which would have been appropriate at
the time of such a precipitating cause may also be indicated
if lasting benefit is to be obtained, since such an event may
still be causing an energy imbalance. A detailed family history is also important in this connection because it may
point to the need of a particular class of homoeopathic
remedies – the nosodes – to counteract an inherited tendency or tendencies.

In the history of the present complaint, detailed eluci-
dation of the various symptoms is necessary, and this is
where many of the strange, probing questions come in.
The homoeopathic doctor is interested in three categories
of symptoms which are termed in homoeopathic parlance
the particular symptoms, the general symptoms, and the
strange, rare and peculiar symptoms.

The particular symptoms are the local symptoms related
to the patient's immediate complaint and are usually the
ones the patient will tell the doctor about first. They are
the complaints the patient will refer to as 'mine' – the 'my'
symptoms: 'my pain', 'my sore stomach', 'the queer sensation in my foot' and so on. It is necessary to characterize
these symptoms as accurately as possible for a good remedy
match. For example, it is not sufficient for the patient to
say that he or she has a headache. The site of the pain –
left- or right-sided, front or back, localized or generalized,
and whether it radiates to anywhere else – and the nature of
the pain – for instance, sharp or dull, piercing, shooting,
stabbing, pounding, throbbing, bruising, cutting, aching
or burning – must be established. The modalities of the
symptom, that is, any conditions which modify it either for
better or worse, such as warmth, cold, movement, rest,

different types of weather, different times of day or even different seasons of the year, may also be vital in selecting the remedy.

More important, however, from the homoeopathic point of view, are the general symptoms of the illness, the 'I' symptoms – the complaints of which the patient says 'I feel' or 'I am' restless, anxious, exhausted or whatever it may be. These symptoms lie at a deeper level than the first class, the particulars, which are localized to the part affected. The general symptoms are experienced by the patient's entire being and give an indication of how the patient as a whole reacts to the illness and to the environment, and of how the body has mobilized its defences in its effort to re-establish harmony and health. These symptoms are characteristic of patients as a whole: whether they are warm- or cold-blooded, how they are affected by temperature or weather, if they sweat unduly, any changes in the emotional or mental state, changes in sleep pattern, preferred position for sleeping, types of dreams, cravings and aversions to particular foods or disorders arising from eating particular foods, and so on. If the patient is female, aggravations or alleviations coinciding with the menstrual cycle, or changes in temperament at particular phases of the menstrual cycle, can also be of value.

The patient's basic emotional and mental characteristics are also of considerable importance in choosing the appropriate remedy. The doctor wishes to know if the patient is usually relaxed or nervous and highly-strung, introverted or extroverted, shy or outgoing, aggressive, weepy, impatient, irritable, hurried, anxious, jealous, suspicious, sensitive, sympathetic, better or worse for sympathy, for company or for being alone, whether he or she bottles up problems or likes to talk about them, or has any overriding fears, for instance of heights, thunder, crowds, strangers, open spaces, enclosed places, the dark, being alone, or death. All this contributes to the general picture of the patient and can often suggest the indicated remedy.

Such detailed discussion of the patient's problems also helps to put the patient at ease, as he or she feels that the doctor is genuinely interested in the complaint and is not dismissing it as trivial or fanciful. This rapport may encourage the patient to mention deeper problems such as sexual or marital difficulties which might not otherwise have been mentioned but which may be important in the overall assessment and treatment of the condition.

The third category of symptoms with which the homoeopathic practitioner is concerned are those which are termed strange, rare or peculiar – symptoms which are *not* characteristic of the illness. For instance, a patient who is chilled but who wishes to remain uncovered and even likes to be fanned; or conversely, a patient with a fever who wishes to be well tucked up with several layers of blankets; burning pains which are relieved by heat; or a patient with a raging temperature who is *not* thirsty. Other examples of strange, rare and peculiar symptoms are sweating on uncovered parts only, a feeling that the limbs are brittle or made of glass, a feeling of being two people, often in conflict, or a feeling that some living creature is jumping about inside the abdomen.

At the end of the consultation, the homoeopathic practitioner has compiled a considerable amount of information about the patient, and it is obvious that such an interview requires considerably longer than is usually experienced with the average general practitioner. The patients also have an opportunity to talk fairly extensively about their problems and how they affect them, and about many aspects of their personalities and personal lives which are not normally touched upon. Any physical examination which the doctor may carry out is similar to that conducted by orthodox physicians, but may be somewhat more detailed.

On the basis of the information thus obtained, the homoeopathic practitioner makes a decision as to the remedy, or possibly remedies, which the patient may require. The process of finding the correct remedy is made easier for the doctor by consulting the many reference manuals which link the symptoms described by the patient to remedies which have these features. More recently much of this information has been put on to computer programs and difficult cases may often be more speedily worked out using this modern technique.

In acute cases the symptoms are usually more outstanding and clear-cut than in chronic cases and remedy selection for acute conditions is usually fairly rapid and straightforward. The majority of acute complaints can be covered with a small group of remedies, many of which are included in the home remedy kit (see Chapter 10 and Appendix 1).

If enough information has been gathered at the first visit, subsequent visits can be quite brief. In the long run, time spent on the first consultation is well worth the effort for both doctor and patient if clear guide-lines are laid for future management. If the doctor succeeds in selecting the correct remedy, many complaints which the patient may have had for many years may be cleared up, so that much time can be saved in the future. Effective therapy also enhances the patient's quality of life and gives the doctor greater job satisfaction. It can therefore give both patient and doctor a feeling of well-being, often on both physical and mental levels.

The practitioner may finish the consultation by explaining to the patient how the remedies are given and how they are to be taken. Homoeopathic remedies are administered in different ways depending on whether the condition being treated is acute or chronic and on the potency, or strength, being used. In acute conditions the remedies are usually used in a high potency and may be given frequently (every five or ten minutes at first) and then at longer and longer intervals (half an hour, one hour, two hours) as the condition improves. In chronic cases, on the other hand, a single dose of a high potency, or a split single dose – that is, three powders to be taken four-hourly – is the usual routine, and this may not be repeated for a month or even longer, depending on the patient's progress. Where a low potency is used, however, this may be prescribed in the form of tablets, one to be taken two or three times a day for a period of two to three weeks or even longer, again depending on the progress made.

It is also explained that the homoeopathic medicines are absorbed from the mouth and that they should be taken with the mouth clean and at a time well spaced from food, drinks or cigarettes. Washing them down with a drink of water should be avoided as this will not allow them to remain in the mouth long enough for absorption to be complete.

It is advisable to store the remedies where they will not be subjected to strong light or sunlight, or to extremes of heat or cold. They should also be kept well away from strong-smelling substances such as camphor or peppermint. This is because heat, light and substances with powerful smells have been found to destroy the power of the remedies. In other words don't keep them on a sunny windowsill next to the mothballs!

Some practitioners also suggest that patients keep off strong tea or coffee over the period of treatment. While there is no overall agreement on this point, if you do consume large amounts of tea or coffee it is advisable, even on general health grounds alone, to reduce your intake if you can.

CHAPTER THREE

WAYS IN WHICH

DOCTORS COME

INTO HOMOEOPATHY

Although homoeopathy has been a part of the British National Health Service since its inception in 1948, it has never been taught as an undergraduate subject in any of the medical schools in Britain. If it is mentioned at all to medical students it is in a derogatory fashion, being described as a method of treating patients with incredibly dilute or immeasurable quantities of materials that could have no possible effect on the body. In fact the word 'homoeopathic' has tended to be regarded as synonymous with 'incredibly minute' or even non-existent. No mention is ever made of any of the basic principles of homoeopathy and the undergraduate who has heard of the subject is likely to qualify with an inbuilt prejudice against it which will be difficult for him or her to overcome later on. The same applies to veterinary practitioners, nurses and pharmacists.

Homoeopathy has therefore become a postgraduate study and has to rely for the recruitment of its practitioners on those members of the medical, dental, veterinary and pharmaceutical professions who are open-minded enough to try new approaches. Although homoeopathy is appealing to the lay practitioner, and the number of lay colleges is increasing rapidly in this country at the present time, such developments are viewed askance by some of the medically qualified practitioners mainly because they fear that lay homoeopaths will not possess an adequate grasp of basic medical principles – a fear reflected in the recent BMA report on alternative medicine. Homoeopathy is not a system of treatment in itself. It is simply one approach to the use of medicinal substances and its place should be firmly within the medical profession as a further tool available to the doctor, dentist or veterinary practitioner in addition to his or her orthodox knowledge. The rise of the lay colleges at the present time is largely the fault of the medical profession itself, a result of its consistent disregard for this approach to treatment so that the demand for it far outweighs the practitioners available to supply that demand.

However, despite the lack of knowledge on the subject, and the prejudices engendered against it, a small but steady stream of doctors is willing to investigate it. There are a number of ways in which they might become interested in the subject.

● Firstly, there is an interest in the subject from an early age if one of the practitioner's own parents, or a close relative, is a homoeopathic practitioner. Such a doctor would have an informed knowledge of the subject before coming into contact with any prejudicial remarks.

● Second, there is personal experience of homoeopathy through having been treated by a homoeopathic doctor, or through having had a member of the family so treated, and being impressed by the results. Chamomilla, which is almost specific for the fractious, teething infant, is probably responsible for more recruits to the homoeopathic cause than any other remedy, even the injury remedy arnica. The relief that chamomilla can bring to the parents, to say nothing of the baby, after a succession of sleepless nights and frantic days has encouraged a number of medical practitioners to look further into this system of therapeutics.

● A third way in which doctors may become interested in homoeopathy is through having one of their patients helped by it when they themselves had failed. Such an experience may encourage the doctor in question to attend a course in homoeopathy to see if it deserves further study.

● Another way in which doctors may be encouraged to investigate the claims of homoeopathy is through an increasing anxiety about the possible toxic side-effects of orthodox pharmaceutical preparations. Such side-effects seem to be becoming increasingly common these days, and many patients are becoming disgruntled with these drugs and are seeking safer alternatives.

● A fifth avenue is that of serendipity, where a doctor comes across homoeopathy purely by chance. This may be in the course of a meeting on alternative methods of therapy which the practitioner may have attended either out of a vague general interest or out of disenchantment with the results of orthodox treatments.

Disenchantment with orthodox approaches is, in fact, bringing a number of new recruits to homoeopathy at the present time. Both the members of the medical profession and their patients are becoming increasingly frustrated by the inability of conventional methods to solve the mounting problem of chronic disease. Advice like 'it's your age' or 'you'll just have to learn to live with it' is beginning to wear thin and many people are seeking desperately for alternatives which hold out the promise of improved health.

In the past few years, a number of magazine articles and television programmes have brought homoeopathy to the attention of the public at large, both to patients and to their health care professionals. Public opinion in general is turning to a more natural approach both to the environment and to health as a reaction to the increasingly mechanized view of man and society which has been developing throughout the greater part of this century. Homoeopathy fits comfortably into a more natural, ecological view of the individual and the society in which he lives. With its emphasis on the importance of personal uniqueness, it gives to the individual a value one is increasingly in danger of losing in this computer age. A feeling of personal importance, a valid place in the overall scheme of things and an appreciation that the material plane does not encompass all there is to life is essential if true health and well-being are to be attained.

Personal experience of Dr Robin Gibson

My own experience with homoeopathy embodies a number of the ways in which doctors can become interested in this subject. It was during my first year at university that I first came across it in a book by James Tyler Kent in a public library. *The Repertory of the Homoeopathic Materia Medica* presented me with a view of patients and diseases which was quite unlike anything which I had encountered, and gave many lively examples of the ways in which Kent had solved the clinical problems with which he had been faced.

Later on in my undergraduate career I was lucky enough to be given some teaching by Dr Douglas Ross, consultant in Glasgow, and had personal experience of the efficacy of homoeopathy when he cured the gingivitis (inflammation of the gums) which had been plaguing me for three weeks with a homoeopathic preparation of mercury. This reinforced my interest in the subject, but as I soon became involved in postgraduate studies in busy medical, surgical and then paediatric units I had little time to pursue it at that stage.

My first practical experience in the use of homoeopathic

remedies was in the treatment of a child with croup. By that time I was working as a registrar in an infectious diseases hospital and had been called out to see a very ill child who had just been admitted to the unit. The standard treatment at that time was to put the child in a steam tent, as this helped the breathing, and if necessary to give an antibiotic, or even cortisone, should there be no improvement with the steam tent. On occasion it was vital in a really bad case to carry out a tracheostomy – that is, to put a small tube into the trachea or windpipe, below the level of the swelling which is causing the breathing difficulty – but this was only rarely required.

I took in with me to the hospital some homoeopathic remedies which are specifics in cases of croup, namely aconite, spongia and *Hepar sulphuris*. When I saw the child at 11 p.m. he was very distressed and restless and matched the remedy picture of aconite. The probable cause in this child's case was a viral infection. The nurses carried out the usual steam tent preparations while I gave the child one dose of aconite. I then went to see three other patients and returned to review the child about twenty minutes later to find him totally at peace and asleep, with no evidence of any respiratory problem. He was discharged two days later with no recurrence. About four days later a similar child was admitted with identical symptoms of croup. He too responded within minutes to the same remedy – aconite. Both the nurses and I were impressed by the speed of action of the remedy, and this experience stimulated me to look into homoeopathy more seriously.

I studied homoeopathy in both Glasgow and London and then started a part-time appointment at the Glasgow Homoeopathic Hospital, taking over in addition a small general practice. This gave me the opportunity of using homoeopathy in a general practice setting, while at the same time dealing with more chronic cases at the hospital where we had a consultant gynaecologist, an ENT surgeon and a consultant general surgeon, each operating once a week. At that time we also ran a children's hospital, so that I had the opportunity of seeing the effects of treatment on acute surgical cases, both pre- and post-operatively, as well as dealing with some fairly ill children and a good mix of diagnostic and management problems in the adult unit. All in all it was a wide variety of clinical situations in which to assess the efficacy of homoeopathic treatment.

My usual practice when visiting a patient with an acute febrile illness was to leave a prescription for the appropriate conventional drug (usually an antibiotic), while at the same time administering the most appropriate homoeopathic remedy with the advice to the patient – or the parents, if the patient was a child – to continue to take the homoeopathic remedy but that if there was no improvement in two to four hours then to take the conventional drug. In the majority of cases the homoeopathic remedy appeared to work effectively and it was rare for the patient to require the conventional therapy.

Chronic disease was a different matter, but gradually I was able to help a number of problem cases which had failed to benefit from conventional treatment. One of the cases which made a deep impression early on in my homoeopathic career was the thirty-two-year-old male patient with the enlarged spleen whose story is presented in Chapter 1. Meanwhile I was consistently impressed by the speed with which our surgical patients recovered following operation, and with the fact that very seldom did we have to catheterize our female patients after gynaecological operations. This procedure of catheterization, that is, of passing a tube into the bladder to relieve a retention of urine, is a not infrequent occurrence in conventional units after such operations. The remedies used most frequently to relieve urinary retention are causticum and staphisagria.

Following this period in the homoeopathic hospital I worked for two years in a professorial immunological unit where I set up studies in allergy to assess the efficacy of homoeopathic remedies in house-dust-mite allergy and hay fever (allergy to grass pollens). This study showed that the homoeopathic remedies were an extremely effective way of managing many patients who had failed to respond to conventional therapies. Later on, as a consultant at the Glasgow Homoeopathic Hospital, I organized two trials in rheumatoid arthritis at the Centre for Rheumatic Diseases. Again it was apparent that the remedies were more effective than conventional therapy alone, often allowing the conventional drugs to be reduced or discontinued.

My continuing experience with homoeopathy serves to confirm the initial impressions that this approach to treatment is a valuable addition to the range of possible treatments available to the doctor (the armamentarium). While it certainly cannot be claimed to be a panacea for all ills, and no system of therapeutics has yet turned out to be that, it is an approach which I would not like to be without. It is applicable to a wide range of patients and their complaints, and its main limitations are in all likelihood the limitations of the practitioner himself.

Personal experience of Dr Sheila Gibson

My own interests have always been in the field of research. After qualifying in medicine and completing my house-officer training, I was employed as a research assistant in a university department of medicine investigating various aspects of lead poisoning. With my husband's increasing involvement with homoeopathy, I viewed with interest the impressive, but off-putting, tomes which contained the gems of homoeopathic philosophy and materia medica, but had no enthusiasm for taking up yet another area of study, and particularly not one as arduous as homoeopathy. I was sympathetic towards the subject and not averse to carrying out some research in that field if the opportunity arose but had no intention of studying it myself.

About four years after completing my work with lead poisoning I became a lecturer in medical genetics, working part-time as by then I had two young children. The post was very interesting and involved a good blend of research, teaching and clinical work. Time and again, however, I recognized the helplessness of the medical profession in the face of most of the genetic problems which I encountered and wondered if there were not some way in which more effective treatments for these diseases could be found.

Both my husband and myself were members of a number of societies dealing with para-medical subjects such as hypnosis, dowsing[1] and radionics,[2] and through these we came to hear about psionic medicine (see Chapter 10). After a homoeopathic meeting which we had attended in London, we went to visit a psionic practitioner in the southern counties to learn a little more about this subject. I was impressed when I discovered that as well as the usual homoeopathic remedies, psionic practitioners used potencies of DNA (deoxyribonucleic acid)[3] and RNA (ribonucleic acid).[4] DNA is the genetic material, the substance of our genes, and RNA is involved in the transfer or transformation of the inherited characteristics into protein synthesis. In other words, RNA is essential for the physical manifestation of the inherited potential of DNA.

I felt that perhaps here, at last, was the way into the treatment of genetic disorders for which I had been searching. I was advised that before studying psionic medicine it would be appropriate to learn homoeopathy and this I duly did, leaving my post in the genetics department for one in the homoeopathic hospital. As my husband was then a consultant there, and involved in research in rheumatology, it was only natural that I joined him in the research field.

It would seem that whenever one begins to explore new territory, more and more inviting vistas open up before one, and more and more interesting and possibly beneficial treatments come one's way. The research currently carried out in the Glasgow Homoeopathic Hospital embraces a number of fields other than homoeopathy, such as diets and diet therapy, neural therapy, magnetic field therapy and acupuncture.

Although it has confidently been predicted by a number of high-ranking orthodox medical practitioners that any research in homoeopathy would rapidly discredit the whole subject, I have not found this to be the case. The more one looks at it, the more interesting this field becomes, both in its applications and in its wider implications for medicine as a whole. Much current research in quantum physics, immunology and genetics seems to come together in the ultimate basis of homoeopathy and helps to throw light on what has until recently been an inexplicable mystery. The further development of these lines of thought may lead to a deeper understanding of the underlying principles of health and disease and an enhanced ability to convert the latter to the former.

CHAPTER FOUR

BACKGROUND

OF HEALTH AND

DISEASE

Before we go too deeply into the treatment of illness with homoeopathy, it is useful to consider in some detail the nature of health and disease, and what is likely to have happened when an individual becomes ill. This is even more important in the case of homoeopathy than in the case of conventional medicine, because without an understanding of the different levels and aspects of the living being it is difficult to appreciate the differences in attitude between homoeopathy and the conventional approach. Moreover, a clear idea of the processes involved is essential for the formulation of a truly beneficial therapy.

Many people these days have a rather negative concept of health in that they tend to look on it as a state in which one does not feel ill or has no pain – in other words, a state of absence of illness. A useful minimal definition is that given by the World Health Organization that 'Health is a state of complete mental, physical and social well-being, and not merely the absence of disease.' Even this is an understatement because true health is a positive, dynamic state in which the individual experiences a feeling of well-being, and is full of energy, enthusiasm, joy and creativity. Such a state tends to be rare in contemporary western civilization.

One of our basic problems is that modern scientific medicine and the society which it serves have to a great extent forgotten who and what human beings are. We tend to view ourselves as physical beings only and to deny that we have anything in the way of a soul or spirit. This leads to the notion that we are nothing more than chemical and mechanical devices, albeit extremely complex and wonderfully integrated ones. We thus tend to think of ourselves as machines, and when things go wrong treatment is organized along similar lines as it is for our machines – servicing, repairing and patching as dictated by the appearance of aches, pains and loss of function. Patients who feel vaguely unwell but for whom no specific diagnosis can be made and who therefore are difficult or impossible to patch or repair tend to be regarded either as malingerers or psychosomatic problems – with the term psychosomatic being equated with unreal or imaginary. This view of the body as a machine and little more has led to the increasing use of pharmaceutical drugs to counteract symptoms and to increasingly sophisticated surgical techniques to remove and replace diseased tissues and organs. The pinnacle of this endeavour currently is transplant surgery or 'spare-part' surgery, analogous to the replacement of worn-out parts in a machine! But are our bodies and our selves truly nothing more than highly complex, sophisticated machines?

In the non-living worlds, the worlds of chemistry and mechanics, systems tend to move from a state of order to a state of disorder – in other words, they tend to break down and disintegrate. We all know this because our cars, television sets, washing machines and refrigerators tend to stop functioning and require servicing and repair, and our houses, if we neglect them, fall into a state of disrepair.

Living systems, on the other hand, do not normally show this tendency. On the contrary they tend to move from a state of relative disorder to one of greater order. Consider any form of life: how it starts as a single cell and grows and develops, with the specialization of different groups of cells to form tissues such as the supporting and connecting substances of the body and organs like the heart or liver. These grow and mature until it becomes a flower, a tree, a tiger or a human being – or whatever it is destined to become – depending on the characteristics transmitted to it through its inherited material, the genes, which are grouped together in its chromosomes.

Or again, take the multitudinous array of chemical substances that exist in the natural world. All of them ultimately start out as two very simple molecules, carbon dioxide and water. Green plants have the marvellous capacity to harness the sun's energy by means of their chlorophyll (the substance which gives them their green colour) to split the water molecule into its component elements, hydrogen and oxygen. They then combine the hydrogen with carbon dioxide to form sugars and release the oxygen into the atmosphere. This is the source of the oxygen which we all require and which we take in when we breathe. Without the oxygen produced from water by green plants, life as we know it on this planet would be impossible. The sugars formed by combining the hydrogen with the carbon dioxide are then converted into substances called starches (the main components of flour and potatoes) which can be elaborated further into the many complex materials which make up the bodies of living things. We tend to take plants for granted, seeing them as just another aspect of the environment and failing to appreciate the vital service which they perform both for ourselves and for all other living creatures on this planet.

It is only when a living organism dies that it becomes subject to the laws of the non-living world, and disintegrates into simpler and simpler molecules or components. The difference between a living organism and one just newly dead is that something which we call life has departed, something which we can neither see, hear, smell, touch, weigh or in any physical sense quantify, but which animates and directs the physical organism while it is alive, and gives it the power to counteract the forces of disintegration and decay.

It should therefore be obvious that the various physical and chemical components of our bodies do not constitute life. They are the tools through which life manifests and functions on the material plane, but without the animating principle – the life force or vital energy – they are nothing more than complex chemistry. They are not capable of organizing themselves in a directional, creative manner. That controlling function is an attribute of the life force, and when that is withdrawn at death the whole complex biochemical organization falls into decay. At the same time the sensory awareness of the organism, and its ability to react to stimuli, are also withdrawn. The person or the animal is just not there any more, although their tissues for the time being may not be biochemically different. Consideration of these facts should be enough to alert us to the possibility that the totality of our being may be much more than just the physical body, and that we may not be in any sense only machines.

Certainly the physical part of our being is the most obvious and no one denies its existence. It is, however, not all that we are because we know that we also have feelings and emotions. Such experiences as love, hate, anger, sympathy, guilt, joy, sorrow and so on are considered to be abstract things as opposed to concrete objects like stones, trees or physical bodies. These abstract entities cannot be seen, smelt, touched or heard, although the effects which they produce on our physical beings can be observed in these ways.

In addition to the emotional plane, we also have a mental sphere. These mental abilities fall into two groups. On the one hand we have the capacity for logical, rational thought

with the ability to deduce or work out solutions to problems, and the analytical powers of scientific inquiry. This
is the scientific and technological side of the mind. On the
other hand we also have the ability to remember past events
and situations, to visualize these and to create in our imagina-
tions future possibilities. Along with this imaginative,
inspirational side of the mind goes the capacity – better
developed in some than in others – for intuition. This is the
imaginative, artistic and intuitive side.

These two aspects of mental function have been related
to the left and right sides (or hemispheres) of the brain,
with the left hemisphere in most people being associated
with the logical, rational, deductive, analytical abilities and
the right hemisphere being associated with the intuitive,
perceptive, imaginative powers. Since, in most people, the
principal speech centres are located in the left hemisphere,
speech is a function of rational, logical thought. The right
hemisphere is largely non-verbal, though right-sided
speech centres are better developed in women than in men.
The right hemisphere functions, therefore, tend to be expressed in terms of symbols and concepts rather than
verbally, which explains why such concepts can be very
difficult to express in words. It is impossible to present
right-brain concepts as reasonable or understandable to
people who have suppressed the greater part of their right-
brain abilities and function virtually entirely in the left-
brain approach.

This concept of the division of our mental attributes into
two quite separate aspects brings us to the frontiers of the
fourth plane of our being, the spiritual level or plane. The
left-brain functions of logical, rational, concrete thought
are directed towards the outer, objective world of physical
reality – the finite, material, worldly plane of existence.
The right-brain functions on the other hand – the perceptive, intuitive, artistic abilities – are directed towards the

inner, subjective world of transcendental reality, a world not bound by space or time but which is infinite and eternal – the spiritual realm as opposed to the material, physical realm. The physical link between the two sides of the brain, known as the *corpus callosum*, has the ability to transfer information from one side to the other, so that the two aspects of mental function should not operate in isolation, but potentially have the capacity for interaction and interplay.

In the left-brain-dominated societies of the west, the value of the right-brain functions are severely questioned and are often dismissed as being outmoded and irrelevant. Extreme positions, however, whether of the right or left brain, are unbalanced, out of harmony and therefore potentially unhealthy. In a well-balanced individual, both aspects should be equally, or roughly equally, developed and we suppress or deny either aspect at the risk of reducing our quality of life.

Some of the relationships associated with the two sides of the brain are illustrated in Figure 1.

The human being, therefore, can be visualized as being composed of at least four different levels or planes: the physical plane, the emotional plane, the mental plane and the spiritual plane – all of which are interdependent and interpenetrating. The principle which animates these planes – holds them together and establishes communication between them – can be visualized as the life force or vital force, the Prana of the Hindus, or the Ch'i energy of the Chinese, that elusive something which departs at death.

In books dealing with the more spiritual aspects of man, the levels are often portrayed as being outside each other, each ascending level being larger than the one below, as shown in Figure 2. The emotional, mental and spiritual levels form an energy field around the body known as the

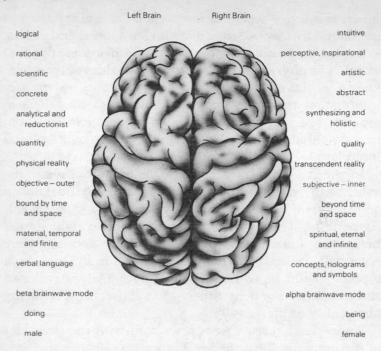

Left Brain   Right Brain

Left Brain	Right Brain
logical	intuitive
rational	perceptive, inspirational
scientific	artistic
concrete	abstract
analytical and reductionist	synthesizing and holistic
quantity	quality
physical reality	transcendent reality
objective – outer	subjective – inner
bound by time and space	beyond time and space
material, temporal and finite	spiritual, eternal and infinite
verbal language	concepts, holograms and symbols
beta brainwave mode	alpha brainwave mode
doing	being
male	female

Figure 1. The relationships of the left and right sides of the brain

aura, aspects of which can be seen by some people and which have recently been partially demonstrated by modern technology. In his book, *The Science of Homoeopathy*, the Greek homoeopathic practitioner Vithoulkas[1] presents a slightly different diagram in which each ascending level is shown as being within and higher than the previous one, with all of them interpenetrated by the life force. He, however, shows only three levels – the physical, emotional and mental – and does not include the spiritual level. This way of representing the four levels is shown in Figure 3. The difference between Figures 2 and 3 is probably not important, each being just a different representation of what can only be a pale reflection of the true state of affairs, just

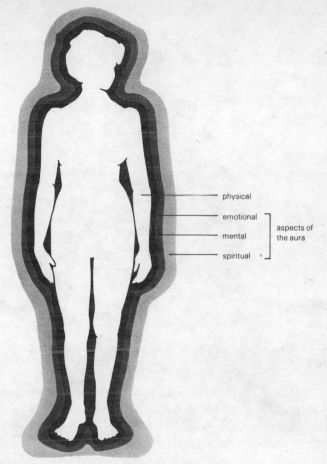

Figure 2. The energy fields of the human being

as any illustration of the body's organs is but a poor reflection of its true inner workings.

That matter is not really as we perceive it has been known to chemists and physicists for over 150 years, but despite Einstein's demonstration, and that of other atomic scientists since, that matter and energy are interchangeable, we persist in our view that physical matter is solid and stable.

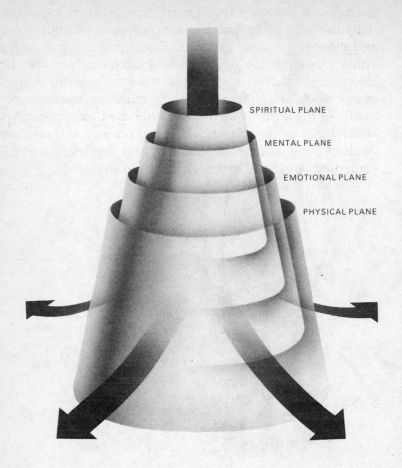

SPIRITUAL PLANE

MENTAL PLANE

EMOTIONAL PLANE

PHYSICAL PLANE

Figure 3. Diagrammatic representation of the energy fields of the human being

But that is only how we perceive it, how it registers itself to our physical senses, and not how it really is.

The building blocks of matter are the atoms which were originally thought to be indivisible. In the last few decades, however, the simple atoms of the early atomic theories have been discovered to be much more complex than was originally thought, and physicists are continually finding more and more sub-atomic particles. These particles may carry either a positive or a negative electrical charge, or may be electrically neutral; some have mass or weight, others appear to be weightless. Different numbers and arrangements of these particles form the hundred or so elements which occur on our planet. Their composition is such that, despite the evidence of our physical senses, they are composed largely of space, as shown in Figure 4.

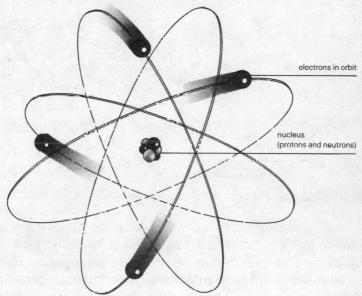

electrons in orbit

nucleus
(protons and neutrons)

Figure 4. Diagram of an atom

Different combinations and arrangements of the atoms form the molecules which range all the way from simple inorganic or non-living compounds like salts, water, oxygen and carbon dioxide to the highly complex organic substances elaborated by living systems and which are essential for their proper functioning. They are produced by life and, though they do not constitute the animating principle, they are essential for the creative energy to manifest and function on the physical plane.

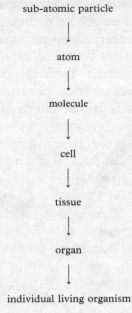

sub-atomic particle

↓

atom

↓

molecule

↓

cell

↓

tissue

↓

organ

↓

individual living organism

Figure 5. Sequence of increasing organization

The increasing complexity of matter forms a series of components of increasing organization as illustrated in Figure 5. The sub-atomic particles are arranged to form the atoms, and different numbers, types and arrangements of atoms form the molecules. As we go up the scale of complexity, many highly evolved and sophisticated molecules are involved in the constitution of even the simplest living cell. The progression from the molecule to the cell is also the leap from the non-living to the living world. With our present-day highly developed technologies, we can re-create many of the complex molecules found in nature, but we cannot create life – another argument in favour of the existence of the life force or life energy, whatever it may be.

Cells organize themselves together to form tissues such as fatty tissue, muscle or bone; tissues organize to form organs, such as the heart, lungs or brain; many organs and tissues, working together, form living bodies, be they plant, animal or human.

This organization and cooperation is to be seen everywhere in nature. Not only do individual cells, tissues and organs integrate and cooperate to form the individual living creature, but individual creatures can cooperate together in sometimes surprising partnerships. We are familiar with the complex societies of the insect world where we see the cooperation of many individuals of the same species to produce the highly organized colonies of the bees, ants and termites. Sophisticated as these are, however, even more remarkable is the interplay between different kingdoms of nature – often, though apparently not always, to the benefit of each.

For instance, sea slugs, a type of mollusc, live in the tidal zones around our coasts and most species are more brightly coloured than the equivalent land slugs which we know so well. They are seemingly helpless creatures,[2] apparently easy prey for fish. The most brightly coloured parts of the sea slug, which therefore attract most attention, are the papillae – hair-like structures which grow from their backs and which have arranged on their surfaces groups of stinging cells known as nettle-cells or nematocysts, which explode at the slightest touch, discharging a barbed, whip-like structure. These cells are believed to function as a defence mechanism against the sea slugs' enemies – fish which would otherwise feed on them.

These nematocysts, however, are not really a part of the sea slug. They are cells derived from animals of the group known as the coelenterates, which includes the sea anemones and jellyfish. These animals possess the nettle-cells or nematocysts, which are arranged near their surfaces, and act as a weapon either of offence or defence for them.

Interestingly enough, sea slugs are able to eat sea anemones without discharging their nematocysts. Even more remarkably, they do not digest the nematocysts along with the rest of the sea anemone, but collect them in their stomachs and then pass them along narrow channels lined by motile hairs which move the contents of the channel in one direction only, and which lead from the stomach to tiny pouches situated near the periphery of the papillae. There the nematocysts are arranged in symmetrical rows, correctly orientated for discharge against the sea slug's enemies. The sea slugs therefore use the defence mechanism of another creature for their own defence.

An example of the interactions between living things in which both partners would appear to benefit equally occurs in the Amazon Forest where one particular species of orchid is pollinated by just one species of bee which seems to be tailor-made to fit the flower which it pollinates. An example of this was shown in a television wild-life programme. The bee enters the flower to collect the nectar, pollinating it in the process, but then finds that it can only escape from the flower by crawling along a narrow, tortuous channel. In the course of this journey of escape, the bee collects the flower's own pollen which pollinates the next flower which the bee visits. The pollination process is so complicated and mechanically wonderful that it is almost beyond belief; and the process is specific for that species of bee and that species of orchid, so that if one partner became extinct, the other would also die out.

These are just two of the many examples which could be quoted of the controlling and interacting forces at work in nature and of the subtle interlinking with occurs throughout the natural world and which maintains the state of order on this planet.

It is difficult to visualize how such intricate and finely tuned mechanisms could have arisen purely by chance, and gradual evolution is unlikely since these instances of cooperation between widely different species appear, in many instances, fully developed, without a series of intermediate forms. The facts, as we perceive them, do suggest the existence of a coordinating intelligence at work behind the scenes, possibly an aspect of that same life energy, or vital force, which we already saw as having an organizing and integrating function in the individual living organism. This life force, which integrates the physical, emotional and mental aspects of the individual, and which is equated here with some part of the spiritual plane, is seen as underlying the whole complex, interlinking and interrelated fabric which is life on this planet.

The scheme of increasing complexity from sub-atomic particle to individual living being yields seven levels of organization, only three of which are in the non-living world. From the level of the cell on, life forces are involved.

Taking ourselves back to our basic physical components, we can say that we are built up from multitudes of particles held together by electrical bonds of varying strengths or intensities. Electrical forces are basic to the system, being attributes of the sub-atomic particles, and it is electrical attraction which holds together the atoms and molecules. Chemical bonds and chemical reactions depend on these electrical forces; all chemical reactions are, in essence, reorganizations of electrical forces, and these continue to be vital at cellular, tissue, organ and total body levels, being manifested in the electrical charges detectable on cell membranes, all the way from simple cells to muscles and nerves. Electrocardiograms (ECGs), electromyograms

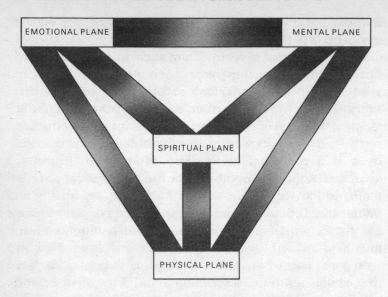

Figure 6. The interrelationships of the energy fields

(EMGs) and electroencephalograms (EEGs) – readings of the electrical activities of the heart, muscles and brain respectively – are aspects of these electrical forces which are essential for the harmonious functioning of the whole body. A living organism can therefore be regarded as an extremely intricate electrical system.

Representing the individual as a series of interpenetrating planes of increasing fineness and subtlety makes it easier to appreciate how changes on any one plane can affect the others. This relationship is illustrated in an alternative fashion in Figure 6. For instance, changes on the physical plane as a result of a toxic substance or an infection can have an effect on the emotional and mental planes. That this does happen is well known. Possibly the commonest example is the post-flu depression that can last for a number of days or even weeks after the physical symptoms of the influenza infection have cleared up. Conversely, stresses on the mental and emotional levels can have an effect on the physical body; for example, duodenal ulcers in executives under pressure or bereavement triggering off rheumatoid arthritis. This was illustrated quite dramatically by a patient who took part in one of our trials on arthritis. Several years before we saw her, she had gone with a friend to visit the war graves in Flanders. Her brother who had been a soldier was killed in Flanders during the Second World War and was buried there. About a month after returning from this trip, she suddenly developed full-blown rheumatoid arthritis.

What effects disturbances on the spiritual plane may have on our mental, emotional or physical well-being are more difficult to assess but it is not impossible that our view of ourselves as machines, with a denial of any spiritual aspect and a consequent loss of meaning in our lives, may be one cause of much of the unhappiness and frustration seen today with results as different as vandalism and cancer – aspects of destruction at one level or another.

The idea of the individual being composed of different interpenetrating and interdependent layers or planes also emphasizes how artificial the distinction is between mental and physical illness. Most illnesses probably contain elements of both, but with a preponderance of one or the other which allows us to classify them accordingly. To do so, however, may cause us to miss the basic underlying reason for the patient's problem. For instance, some years ago a patient came to the out-patient department complaining of severe bouts of depression. He had suffered from these for seven years and had been in and out of mental hospitals many times and had received every available treatment including electro-convulsive therapy (ECT) – all to no avail. Homoeopathy did not help him either but at his third visit he commented that he did not know which came first, his sinus problem or his depression. The mention of a sinus problem suggested a possible allergy and he was put on a simple allergy-exclusion diet consisting of lamb, pears and water for five days. This improved both his sinus problem and his general health. He then began adding back one food per day and when he included instant coffee it produced another bout of severe depression. He then remembered that seven years previously an instant coffee machine had been installed in the building where he worked and he had fallen into the habit of having a cup every time he passed it. He was advised to cut out all instant coffee from his diet and since then has kept very well by doing so.

Health, as we have said, is a dynamic, positive state of well-being, a state of harmony and balance on all levels of existence. Disease is literally dis-ease, a state of disharmony and imbalance on one or other, or more, of these levels. In order to effect a lasting cure, it is necessary to correct the fundamental imbalance or disharmony. It may, however, be difficult to determine what the basic imbalance is.

Consider again the scheme of the different inter-dependent planes of being, interpenetrated by the life force principle. While the organism remains filled with the life force, it can counter the disintegration and decay to which the non-living world is subject. A living being is therefore in essence a potentially self-healing system. We are all well acquainted with that other property of living things – their ability to reproduce themselves. From the humblest virus up to the human level all living things are able to reproduce their kind, an attribute which no machine possesses. Living systems are therefore potentially self-healing and self-replicating. This ability of living things to heal themselves is often amazing. We take for granted our capacity to heal cuts and scratches, knit broken bones and cure colds. We tend to dismiss the ability of a lizard or a salamander to re-grow a lost tail by saying that these are relatively simple and unspecialized creatures. However, dramatic recoveries are not confined to the reptilian world. A recent claim by an accident and emergency consultant in Sheffield[3] that children, and even adults, could regrow their finger tips, providing that the injury did not extend as far as the terminal or end joint, was greeted with considerable scepticism by the medical profession. We do not know of any other reports of a similar nature but we know of a lady whose left hip joint was completely destroyed as a result of rheumatoid arthritis. The hip and femur bones were fused together and no movement was possible at that joint. However, within six months of our treating her, she had regrown a new hip joint. X-ray appearances and function are now both markedly improved despite the fact that it is generally believed that once joint cartilage (the substance lining the joint space) has been destroyed it can never be regenerated.

Another interesting case is that of a little boy who had had a difficult birth and had been left slightly spastic. When seen at the age of six, he had poor muscle control and could not fasten up his buttons or tie his shoe-laces. He also found learning at school a trial. Since lack of coordination was a major factor in his problem, a modified form of acupuncture which can correct a disturbed energy flow was used in this case. Within a few minutes of this treatment being given, he was able to button up his coat. Now, after two or three treatments, his coordination has improved and he is also doing much better at school.

This method of acupuncture is also of value in over 60 per cent of cases of multiple sclerosis. We now have many multiple sclerosis patients who have benefited from this treatment which is well illustrated by one of our early cases. This was a man of forty-six who had had multiple sclerosis for six years. He had had a spell about two years previously when he had been in a wheel-chair for a few weeks, but had managed to get himself out of it and stagger around with two tripods. When first seen at the homoeopathic clinic, he was just able to get around with one tripod. Within minutes of being given the treatment his walking was much improved, and the following day he was walking around without any sticks and was also able to climb up and down stairs unaided – a thing he had been unable to do for at least two years. Repeated treatments as required keep him on his feet.

Disease, as we have already said, is basically a state of imbalance or disharmony. The insults or stresses which cause the imbalances and so give rise to disease can be of two types:

• Noxious or harmful stimuli attacking the organism from without – from the outside environment. Examples of such stresses are injuries, infections and toxic substances entering the body; emotional stresses such as bereavement, disappointment and frustration; social and mental pressures such as guilt, work-load deadlines and so on. All these can cause a stress on the body and if they are stronger than the body's power to withstand them, then imbalances will be caused, initially at the level under stress.

• Imbalances arising from within – the inherited tendencies. The most obvious examples of these are the inherited genetic diseases such as phenylketonuria, muscular dystrophy, or haemophilia, but genetic factors play a part in most, if not all, diseases.

Chronic degenerative diseases result from a combination of external environmental factors and internal inherited factors, with the proportion due to each varying both with the individual and the disease.

The body's first line of protection against environmental stimuli is effected through the defence or immune system. This is composed of white blood cells, the leucocytes, and various blood-borne and tissue factors – the different classes of antibodies. Initially thought to be simple, continuing research in immunology has revealed that this system is extremely complex and under stringent control through a series of checks and feedbacks. It is specifically aimed at inactivating and destroying invading infectious agents (bacteria, viruses and other parasites) and with neutralizing some types of toxins (poisons). Interlinked with the immune system is the hormonal or chemical messenger system, some aspects of which (adrenaline, released in excess in fight, flight and fright situations) come into play in reactions to emotional and mental stress, and other aspects of which are concerned with controlling healing and repair.

In the last two decades a whole new system of checks and balances – the prostaglandin system – has been discovered. The prostaglandins are messenger molecules whose role is to harmonize the many complex biochemical reactions which occur within cells, and to integrate the individual cells one with another. The prostaglandins also set off or cut down or stop specific enzyme reactions within the cells, thus allowing the body to react to the environmental stresses and insults and so keep itself intact. The prostaglandins are usually manufactured at the site where they are needed and are short-lived molecules, being very quickly destroyed. They are thus transient and are present in trace amounts only in any one situation and at any one time. It would seem that they are the molecules responsible for maintaining the harmonious, smooth running of the body's many functions, stimulating the release of hormones when required, organizing healing and repair and bringing into play the complex workings of the immune system. The success of the body in maintaining its integrity or its wholeness therefore depends on a highly intricate series of interlinked specific reactions and responses.

In the development of illness, therefore, a combination of external and internal factors is involved in the majority of cases in the production of the original imbalance, and this imbalance can occur on any level, depending on the main thrust of the external stress. The body, however, being a potentially self-healing system, will combat the effects of the imbalance to the best of its ability through the prostaglandin, immune and hormonal systems. In doing so it attempts to limit the effects of the imbalance to the most superficial levels – in other words, the physical level – and only if it fails to do so will emotional imbalances, or if the stresses go deeper, mental imbalances, be manifest. This means that at whatever level the stresses or insults initially attack the system, the effects, if the body is strong enough, will be confined to the physical plane. Of course if the body's self-healing power is stronger than the factors causing the disturbance, it will heal itself completely. It is only when the body's own powers are insufficient to deal with these disturbing factors, that medical intervention becomes necessary.

The fact that the disturbing factors may be complex, and that the body tends to limit the symptoms of disease to the physical plane if at all possible, can make it difficult to determine what the basic underlying imbalance is. The result is that often illnesses are considered to be purely physical when in fact they have an emotional trigger, as in the case of the lady who developed rheumatoid arthritis after her visit to Flanders, or a mental or possibly even spiritual precipitating factor. Conversely, emotional or mental problems can arise from a physical cause, as was the case with the victim of the instant coffee, and this is even less likely to be recognized by orthodox practitioners.

This concept of precipitating factors must always be borne in mind. An individual may be under stress from a variety of factors, possibly both internal and external, but is able to cope and is strong enough to keep the system in balance, but only just. Along may come a sudden additional stress, the last straw on the camel's back, as it were, which could be a disappointment in job prospects or even redundancy, bereavement, a fight with a colleague, or something nasty in last night's curry, and the balance breaks down and illness supervenes. According to the nature and strength of the stress in relation to the body's own reserves, or lack of them, and the individual's inherited constitution, the resulting illness could be a minor gastro-intestinal upset, a severe attack of colitis, a heart attack, rheumatoid arthritis, nervous breakdown and so on. The disease produced is not necessarily obviously related to any discernible precipitating cause, which makes the classification of diseases according to the symptoms and with a known list of causes somewhat meaningless and arbitrary.

In the next chapters we will go on to consider what homoeopathy is, how it arose and developed, and how it fits in with the scheme of health and disease outlined here.

CHAPTER FIVE

WHAT IS

HOMOEOPATHY?

Homoeopathy is not a complete system of medicine but a system of therapeutics – that is, a system of administering drugs. The remedies are derived mainly from the natural world (the mineral, plant and animal kingdoms) and are selected and administered according to a set of basic principles. Doctors using homoeopathy have the same training and basic qualifications as their conventional colleagues, and study homoeopathy as an additional postgraduate subject. Diagnosis is the same whether the doctor is homoeopathic or orthodox, but the homoeopathic doctor has the advantage of not needing a diagnosis before treatment begins, since it is the patient rather than the disease for whom the prescription is made.

The fundamental underlying principle of homoeopathy is that what a remedy can cause in the way of symptoms and signs it can also cure – that is, the principle of treatment by similars. This is the reverse of the conventional approach, which uses its remedies and drugs to counteract the symptoms and signs of disease – in other words, treatment by opposites. So in treatment by similars a remedy which mimics the symptoms and signs of the illness is given to treat the illness; in treatment by opposites the illness is treated with remedies which counteract the symptoms and signs.

Homoeopathy also differs from the orthodox approach in that it concentrates on the body's own inherent ability to heal itself and aims to work along with this ability, to enhance it where necessary, to seek out the basic underlying causes of an illness and to effect where possible a permanent cure. Thus homoeopathy seeks to restore the organism to harmony and balance. Orthodox medicine, on the other hand, tends to view the body as a machine and uses its drugs and remedies to counteract the symptoms and signs of an illness. It therefore tends to be palliative rather than curative. In the orthodox view the illness is considered to be the sum total of the symptoms and signs which it produces.

In homoeopathy a rather different view is taken. It is considered that when an individual becomes ill, that is, out of balance, the organism reacts in a way which attempts to restore the balance, that is, curatively. This reaction produces the symptoms and signs which the patient feels and the doctor can observe. The symptoms and signs are not considered to be the illness but rather to be the results of the body's reaction to the original state of imbalance. They thus become an indicator of how far out of balance the organism is and of how deeply the system has been affected, and are specific to the individual irrespective of the basic cause of the imbalance. They can therefore be used in designing the treatment required to restore the individual to balance and hence to health.

Because individuals vary, their responses to the same stress or insult may also vary, which means that treatment has to be prescribed specifically for that patient. For instance, a patient with influenza might feel very chilly, restless and anxious, want lots of warmth and be thirsty for small sips of cold water. The eyes and nose may be streaming with a watery, excoriating discharge which causes redness and soreness of the upper lip, nose and cheeks. He or she may also have vomiting and possibly diarrhoea. Such a patient would require the remedy *Arsenicum album*. Another person in the same flu epidemic might feel very tired and lethargic, chilly and shivery up the back and with a dull occipital headache. This patient just wants to sit miserably by the fire, warming the back, or to lie tucked up cosily in bed, and does not want to move around or to make any effort whatsoever. This person would require gelsemium. Yet another sufferer in the same epidemic may have a very sore body and feel as if all his or her bones have been broken. This one would be given *Eupatorium perfoliatum*. It is the same influenza virus which has affected all three patients, but their individual reactions to the infection have been different and so their treatment will also be different.

When a part of the body becomes infected the immune system comes into play, rushing white blood cells and immune proteins to the scene of the infection in an attempt to inactivate or kill the invading organisms and to clear up the damage. The site of the infection thus becomes hot, throbbing, swollen and often red – due to the increased fluid and cells present – and painful due to the swelling. The heat, redness, pain and swelling are the classical signs of inflammation and are very obviously the result of the body's reaction to the infection and not the cause of the illness. Another example is the case of a generalized infection in which a fever is often observed – the result of the body's attempt to make the environment unsuitable for the invading organism and so rid itself of it. The fever is therefore the result of the body's reaction to the imbalance or stress – in this case an infecting organism, the influenza virus. A homoeopathic doctor would give a remedy selected to help the body in its fight against the virus – thus working along with the body's healing force; whereas an orthodox doctor might give aspirin or some other drug to bring down the fever – thus, in effect, working against the body's healing force. This difference in approach constitutes the fundamental difference between the homoeopathic and orthodox systems of drug use.

This leads directly to a further difference: an orthodox practitioner is likely to treat all cases of influenza with the same drug, an antibiotic perhaps; whereas the homoeopathic practitioner may use different remedies, depending on the patient's reaction to the influenza, as we saw in the cases illustrated above.

It is one thing to look at an ill person and say that they are out of balance. It is quite another thing to assess how out of balance the individual is and how to set about restoring the balance. The only clues we have are the symptoms and signs, both past and present, and any history there may be of possible precipitating factors. The symptoms and signs are therefore of paramount importance in designing the treatment.

The principle of treatment by similars – that what a remedy could produce it could also cure – was as far as we know first put forward by the Greek physician Hippocrates in the fifth century BC. Over the centuries, however, it was forgotten or disregarded and it was not until the end of the eighteenth century that it was rediscovered empirically by the German physician Samuel Hahnemann. Having discovered that if he took cinchona or Peruvian bark, from which quinine is derived, he developed the symptoms and signs of intermittent fever (malaria), and knowing that cinchona was an effective treatment for malaria, Hahnemann went on to experiment with other substances in use at the time to see what symptoms and signs they would produce. He tried many of them out on himself and on his family and friends, and noted the effects produced by each. He then complemented these observations by giving the appropriate remedy to patients who displayed similar symptoms and signs, and found that he had discovered a therapeutic tool eminently superior to any in use at that time. By experiment and observation, Hahnemann worked out the drug pictures of many remedies and laid down the principles whereby they were to be used – remedies and principles which are still as valid today as they were when Hahnemann first discovered them. He spent the rest of his life adding to his materia medica and developing his ideas about disease and its treatment.

Principles of homoeopathy

● *Treatment of like by like (the similimum principle, or the law of similars):* that what a remedy can cause in the way of symptoms and signs, it can also cure. This is the basic underlying principle of homoeopathy and the one from which its name is derived. To be successful the remedy should match the totality of the patient's symptoms and signs as closely as possible – as demonstrated in the three separate cases of influenza. Another commonly experienced complaint is a sudden fever. For instance, a patient with a fever may be very hot and flushed, with a bright red face, a full bounding pulse, staring eyes with widely dilated pupils, and a burning, hot skin. He or she is better for warmth and dislikes being uncovered. There is often a throbbing headache which is made worse by noise, light or jarring movement, and the patient just wants to lie still in a darkened room, well covered up. Another patient may have a similar fever and be hot and flushed but in this case, although the pulse is bounding, the pupils are not dilated. The onset of symptoms is very sudden and the outstanding ones are anxiety and restlessness and a terrible fear that he or she is going to die. There is an intense thirst and the patient wants to throw off the bedclothes. In the first case the remedy would be belladonna and in the second, aconite. Although both patients have a fever, it is the subtle differences that match the remedy. Obviously, the closer the match, the more successful the treatment.

● *The concept of the provings:* the way in which the drug pictures are built up for each remedy. The remedy is given in different strengths or potencies to groups of healthy volunteers (the provers) over a period of time. The provers note daily in their diaries any symptoms and signs which they develop, any changes in attitude or temperament which they may experience, or any other changes. At the end of the trial period all the diaries are collated, most importance being attached to those effects which were produced in the greatest number of provers. The information gained from such provings is enlarged by adding in any known toxic effects of the remedy in question which may have been noted in cases of poisoning (either accidental or otherwise) and is completed by noting any symptoms and signs which were not observed in the provings but which cleared up unexpectedly in patients given that remedy on the provings indications. In this way a great volume of information has been accumulated on the two to three thousand remedies in the homoeopathic materia medica.

● *The concept of the minimum dose.* Many of the substances which Hahnemann used homoeopathically were known poisons and therefore could not be administered safely to patients in large doses. Moreover, Hahnemann discovered that if a patient needed a particular remedy he or she tended to be very sensitive to it – much more so than someone for whom it was not indicated. He therefore experimented with diluting his remedies in an attempt to find that dose which would still be curative but would not produce unwanted side-effects. His biological tinctures and other soluble substances were diluted in a water/alcohol mixture, using two scales of dilution: the 1 in 10 known now as the D or X (D = decimal, X = 10) range of potencies; and the 1 in 100, the C (C = centesimal) range. Insoluble materials were triturated (ground up) with lactose (sugar of milk) in dilutions of 1 in 10 or 1 in 100. After the third trituration such substances became soluble, and dilution was then continued using the water/alcohol diluent. At each stage of the dilution Hahnemann subjected his solutions to a succession of powerful shocks by bringing the vials in which they were contained down hard several times on to a firm surface. He did this, presumably, to ensure that the solutions were thoroughly mixed before proceeding to the next dilution. This resulted in each solution being subjected to a series of powerful sharp shocks – a process which he termed succussion.

● *The concept of potency.* To his surprise Hahnemann discovered that remedies prepared in this way often became more powerful therapeutic agents than the original starting materials – a purely empirical observation. Moreover, remedies prepared by dilution without succussion did not display this increased therapeutic power. Hahnemann therefore named diluting and succussing his solutions 'potentization', since this process increased the potency or power of the therapeutic agents.

The process of triturition to which insoluble materials were subjected involved grinding one part of the starting material with nine (or ninety-nine) parts of lactose – a sugar which possesses very abrasive crystals. The act of grinding, which could be continued for several hours, resulted in the insoluble starting material being reduced to very small fragments which were distributed on the surface of the lactose particles. When this process was repeated several times the particles of the starting material became so small that the total surface area available for reaction was very great. In the case of a 3X potency the surface area could be increased by a factor of 1000, and by a factor of one million in the case of a 6X potency. Hahnemann found that many substances which were inactive in the crude form became active therapeutic agents when treated in this way.

Although theoretically any potency can be used, in practice it was found that some potencies were more effective than others. In Britain the main potencies used are 1X, 2X, 3X, 6X, 3C, 6C, 12C, 30C, 200C, 1M, 10M, 50M, CM, MM and occasional higher ones. M stands for a thousand, so a 10M potency, for instance, has been diluted 1 in 100, ten thousand times. In Europe a number of other, lower potencies are more often used. In modern homoeopathic pharmacies the succussion process is now carried out by machines.

● *The concept of the single remedy.* This principle follows directly from the principle of the cure by likes. The homoeopathic physician is trying to match his patient to the most like remedy, and it follows that the patient should resemble closely only one remedy at a time. The remedy may change, or in acute injuries more than one remedy may be required, but in classical homoeopathy the remedies are administered one at a time and not as a mixture. This is logical also on the grounds that the remedies were proved as the single remedy and not as mixtures, and mixtures of remedies may have effects which are different from those of their component parts.

Where more than one remedy is required they can be given in sequence, one at a time, a certain length of time apart – one every ten minutes, for example, or one every half hour. Administering the remedies in this way allows the body to process each remedy individually, a situation analogous to presenting a computer with only one program at a time. If one attempted to present a computer with more than one program at a time, it would be unable to deal with the situation and would indicate that an error had been made.

Although the idea that the remedies should be given singly is the classical approach and was advocated strongly by the American physician Dr James Tyler Kent, other approaches, developed particularly in France and Germany, use mixtures of remedies. The doctors in these countries claim that their results are as good as those obtained by giving just one remedy at a time. This is a moot point which requires further study before it can be resolved.

● *The law of the directions of cure:* This was enunciated by Hahnemann's pupil, Dr Constantine Hering, and is of practical use in deciding how a course of treatment is progressing. Hering stated that a cure should proceed: from above, downwards – from the head or upper regions of the body down towards the feet; from within, out – from the internal organs out to the joints or skin; from more important to less important organs – from the liver, heart or lungs out to the joints or skin; from the present backwards in time – going back into the patient's medical history. Hering realized that disease was the result of imbalance somewhere in the body and that if a true cure was to be effected, the imbalance had to be corrected. He visualized it as being brought out from the deeper levels of the individual to the surface and finally dispersed altogether.

If we consider once again the four-fold diagram of the physical, emotional, mental and spiritual planes or levels of the individual – with each plane within and higher than the previous one – we can see the correlation with Hering's directions of cure (Figure 3, p.54). As the disturbance goes more deeply into the organism from the physical to the emotional plane, from the emotional to the mental and finally to the spiritual, it is at the same time becoming higher up in the organism as it is pictured diagrammatically in Figure 3. In bringing out the imbalance, therefore, it should appear in progressively lower and more superficial regions of the body. This idea also correlates with the positions we ascribe to the various functions of the individual in that the physical outer layer is associated particularly with the digestive and generative processes in the abdominal region, emotions are associated with the heart in the thorax and thinking is an attribute of the brain in the head. Therefore, in correcting an imbalance, the effects should ripple out from above, downwards, and from within, out, as Hering observed. The more important organs such as the brain, heart and liver are either high up or deep within the organism, so the direction from more important organs out to less important organs (such as the skin or the peripheral joints) is also in agreement with this model.

Moving from the present backwards in time implies that one can, with patience, go back into a patient's past medical history correcting successive imbalances – rather like peeling an onion layer by layer – until the original, deeply submerged imbalance is uncovered and corrected. That this can be done is borne out in practice, and it is sometimes noted that, in the course of treatment for some long-standing chronic condition, patients will re-experience old symptoms which they may have forgotten about.

An example of this is the case of a lady of forty-five who attended the clinic with neuralgia which had been present for some years. Her main complaint was a severe pain which radiated to the left eyeball. She had a history of aching in the chest, pain extending to both shoulder blades, and neck pain associated with tiredness of both the upper and lower arms and hands. The indicated remedy appeared to be spigelia, but when she was given this she developed palpitations and became quite anxious. Pulsatilla seemed to cover the case as it now presented and successfully treated both the anxiety and the palpitations. It turned out that she had had palpitations in the past but had forgotten about them.

This ability of homoeopathy to go back into a patient's medical history gives it the edge over orthodox drugs which only mask the problem. What can the orthodox practitioner do if a patient tells him that she has never been well since her husband died some ten years ago (grief reaction) or since the dreadful fright she experienced when she had a car crash many years ago? The homoeopathic physician can on the other hand give the appropriate remedies for grief or fright, or whatever else it may have been, and experience the satisfaction of being told that the patient now feels better than she has done for years.

This is illustrated by the case of a girl who experienced a tremendous shock some three to four years before being seen at the homoeopathic out-patient clinic. She had come in from work one evening to find her mother and father dead in each other's arms. She was profoundly upset and had never really recovered from the shock. She felt dazed and was drifting through life never feeling well, sleepless, anxious and just not coping. She was given a high potency of opium which appeared to be the indicated remedy for this numb state. The following day she felt that everything was going very slowly and by the next day she felt that she was back to normal. Her energy and enthusiasm for life returned, her sleep pattern became normal once more and she was able again to cope with life.

Another case is that of a woman who did not cry when her mother died ten years before. She had been very attached to her but for some reason was quite unable to cry over her death. She had never felt well since then. She lacked energy and her emotions were suppressed. She was given *Natrum muriaticum* 10M with no effect. However, this did seem to be the indicated remedy, so she was then given a low potency (3X) twice daily for a period of two weeks. Within a couple of days of taking this, she began to weep, and she then became very concerned because she just could not stop crying. However after two weeks, the weeping cleared up and she felt very much better, back to her old self of ten years before.

These two cases also illustrate the effect that emotional blocks or upsets can have on the overall health of the individual.

A past stress of a different nature is seen in the case of a woman of twenty-seven who had felt chronically debilitated and unwell for years. She had no energy and tended to be listless and lethargic. On taking her history, it was discovered that when she was twelve or thirteen she had had frequent nose bleeds and had lost a great deal of blood. China (cinchona) is a remedy which is indicated in this situation, and when she was given it, she rapidly regained her energy and vitality.

As another illustration there is the interesting case of a lady of seventy. When she was thirty-six, she had had an operation to repair a uterine prolapse. During the operation, unfortunately, one of her ureters (the tube which takes the urine from the kidney to the bladder) was nicked and the surgeon had no option but to transplant that ureter into the bowel. Since then, for thirty-four years, she had lived a fairly unpleasant life as a result of the relocation of the ureter and had to take potassium tablets to prevent her blood potassium level from becoming too low. She was chilly and irritable, liked tasty foods and vinegar, and had an aversion to fat, meat and milk. Sepia is a remedy which has a symptom picture of tiredness, weakness and a dragging down sensation, and often an actual prolapse. The patient is chilly and irritable and finds it difficult to cope. There is usually a desire for vinegar, pickles and tasty foods, and a dislike for fat, meat and milk. The patient's general state as well as her history of prolapse suggested that sepia be given. She rapidly began to feel better and surprisingly she was now able to discontinue the potassium tablets. It would seem that in this case the remedy had corrected a biochemical imbalance.

Hering's concepts are of general value although patients often improve gradually without the directions being too obvious or without any recurrence of old symptoms. However, should there be an apparent worsening of symptoms, Hering's law is useful in assessing whether the symptoms now presenting are part of a previous disease process which has been unmasked transiently during the healing phase or a new, undesirable pattern which is usually treated with another remedy.

If the patient's well-being is enhanced or if a problem such as asthma is cured, but joint pains flare up or a skin rash develops, the physician can reassure the patient that things are moving in the right direction and that the joint or skin problem should be transient and will also clear up in due course.

If, on the other hand, an arthritic patient reported that the joint problems had cleared up but that she was becoming increasingly anxious and irritable, then the physician would be worried and would be certain that the wrong treatment had been given, even though, superficially, it would seem to have been effective.

This happened to a man with eczema and asthma who was treated with a low potency of sulphur which improved both symptoms. That it was the wrong remedy was discovered later when he was given a higher potency which helped the eczema but made the asthma worse. A potency of house dust cleared up this case.

It is therefore important to keep the law of the directions of cure in mind if a thorough and lasting improvement is to be obtained.

● *Repetition of the remedy*. In classical homoeopathy a single dose of a high potency is given to the patient and, assuming improvement, is not repeated for as long as the patient continues to improve. It is only when improvement ceases but further improvement is possible, or the patient begins to deteriorate again, that the dose is repeated, as it appears that the initial dose has been exhausted and more is required. The situation is rather similar to that of pushing a child on a swing. The swing is pushed and is not pushed again until it has come right back to its starting point. If it is pushed at the wrong point of the swinging cycle, the motion is upset and it tends to stop. In a similar way, if a homoeopathic remedy is repeated before it is required, the repetition can upset the efficient working of the remedy and may even undo all the good that has already been done.

Homoeopathic potencies are therefore quite different from conventional drugs which have to be administered daily, and possibly several times a day, over a period of weeks or longer. The low potencies are, however, administered in this way. In the case of the low potencies, that is, those below the 12C potency, material doses, albeit small ones, are present. They are therefore more akin to the conventional drugs.

Other Approaches to Homoeopathy

What has been described so far is basically classical homoeopathy as discovered by Hahnemann and developed further by Kent. Although homoeopathy has survived for close on two hundred years without drastic changes, it is not a static thing, and variations and modifications have been made to it throughout its history. Hahnemann was the first to start modifying what he himself had enunciated and towards the end of his life he developed a further series of dilutions which he called the LM potencies, in which the material was diluted 1 in 50,000 at each step, rather than the more usual 1 in 10 or 1 in 100 dilution steps. The LM series produces very high dilutions and although not greatly favoured is used on occasion.

Another approach to remedy potentization is that devised by Korsakoff. The classical method of potency preparation requires the use of a fresh tube or vial at each dilution stage. In the Korsakoff method, however, just one tube is used. The first dilution is prepared and the tube is then emptied, the amount left being considered to be equivalent to one drop. Nine (or ninety-nine) drops of the diluent are then added and the process is repeated. This method is infinitely more economical of tubes than the classical method and seems to produce effective remedies. Though not used by homoeopathic pharmacies in this country for potencies below the 1M, it is used commercially in Belgium for all potencies, and is also used when a practitioner has to make a specific potency for a particular patient, such as a potency of chloroform for a case of chloroform allergy.

Hahnemann's original remedies were drawn from the mineral, plant and animal kingdoms. However, as he gained experience with his new system of therapeutics, he realized that inherited tendencies lay at the root of many chronic health problems and he developed a further class of remedies, which he called nosodes, to counteract these inherited traits. The nosodes are prepared from disease products such as discharges, the contents of skin vesicles or bacterial or viral cultures. Over the years Hahnemann's original nosodes have been greatly added to and now there are nosodes prepared from all the infectious diseases. A special class are Paterson's bowel nosodes which were prepared from cultures of intestinal bacteria obtained from patients with specific health problems. The nosodes are invaluable for clearing up inherited predispositions and acquired disease toxins which often cannot be treated in any other way.

Similar to the idea of producing remedies from disease processes which can then be used to treat the effects of that disease is the idea of potentizing individual substances to counteract allergies and sensitivities to them. This technique is known as isopathy and is well illustrated by the case of chloroform allergy which was described in Chapter 1. Here, an allergy to chloroform was successfully treated using a homoeopathic preparation of chloroform. Any substance can be converted into a homoeopathic remedy and used in this way. A common example is penicillium, prepared from penicillin, and used to treat cases of penicillin allergy.

We have then in homoeopathy a system of therapeutics which aims at helping the body's innate self-healing abilities by the use of remedies derived in the main from the mineral, vegetable and animal realms. The remedies are prescribed on the basis of the symptoms and signs experienced by the patient and are usually given in the form of homoeopathic potencies. Two methods of preparing the potencies, the Hahnemannian and the Korsakoff, exist and the decision as to whether to use high or low potencies varies with the type of illness present and the prescriber. In general, low potencies are used more extensively in Europe than in Britain, where the whole potency range from low to very high is available to the practitioner.

All aspects of the patient, the emotional, mental and spiritual planes as well as the physical, are taken into consideration in the homocopathic approach to medicine. They are important both from the point of view of the cause of the illness and for matching the remedy to the patient. Therapeutic systems which disregard the more subtle aspects of the individual are likely to miss some at least of the precipitating factors in disease causation and are therefore likely to be less effective in treatment.

CHAPTER SIX

THE HISTORICAL

BACKGROUND

TO HOMOEOPATHY

The basis of homoeopathy is by no means a recent concept. As long ago as the fifth century BC, Hippocrates had stated that there were two methods of treating disease. On the one hand there was treatment by opposites, when a medicament was used to oppose or counteract the symptoms and signs of disease, and on the other hand there was treatment by similars, stimulating healing in the body by giving a substance which would mimic the symptoms and signs of the disease. In treatment by opposites an attack was made on the disease, the seed. In treatment by similars the remedy was used to stimulate the body's own healing powers (the *vis medicatrix naturae* or healing force of nature) thus strengthening the body, the soil.

These two approaches to medical treatment remained in use for several centuries, but by the time of Galen in the second century AD medicine had fallen into a state of chaos. Galen set about systematizing and rationalizing medical thought, and constructed an elaborate theory of the cause and treatment of disease which emphasized the importance of treatment by opposites while treatment by similars was neglected and forgotten. So dogmatic and authoritarian was Galen that his ideas dominated medical thought for many centuries. The medical profession found his theories very difficult to shake off, even when they were demonstrated to be manifestly false. An example of this was the abuse which

Harvey received when he demonstrated the system of blood circulation in the body because what he had discovered was not in accordance with what Galen had said. Thus the idea of treatment by opposites came to dominate medical thought and does so till this day.

Nonetheless this method was not highly successful, and over the centuries more and more heroic practices were introduced in an effort to combat disease. In the sixteenth century the Swiss physician Paracelsus tried to introduce more logical and effective methods of treatment and laid the foundations of a pharmaceutical approach to drug selection, while at the same time reviving the idea of treatment by similars. Even so, by the end of the eighteenth century many medical treatments had become cruel and barbaric, with blood-letting, purges, enemas and ever more complex mixtures of often toxic drugs being the main forms of treatment.

Such was the state of affairs when Dr Samuel Hahnemann appeared on the scene. Hahnemann was born in 1755 in the pottery town of Meissen on the River Elbe in the Electorate of Saxony. His father, his paternal grandfather and one of his uncles were all porcelain painters in the Meissen potteries, but because of the disastrous economic effects of the Seven Years War his family were not well off. Despite financial difficulties, however, Hahnemann displayed such intellectual ability that his teachers helped him in his studies and allowed him to finance his education by tutoring the younger children in the school. A brilliant linguist, he was also deeply interested in botany, chemistry and other scientific subjects. Despite the opposition of his father he took up the study of medicine, first at Leipzig University and then in Vienna, where his funds ran out, forcing him to take employment for a time with the Governor of Transylvania until he had accumulated sufficient money to continue his studies. He finally graduated from the University of Erlangen in 1779 at the age of twenty-four.

He set up in practice in the copper-mining town of Hettstedt but soon discovered that he was out of sympathy with the barbaric medical practices of his time which often showed little compassion for, or understanding of, the patient. Medicine was riddled with superstition and ignorance and Hahnemann had little time for blood-letting, either by venesection or the application of leeches; the violent purges with emetics and enemas, aimed at ridding the body of the disease-producing influences; and the host of concoctions of various substances, many of which, such as arsenic or mercury, were highly toxic. Some of these mixtures contained as many as fifty or sixty different ingredients, and Hahnemann reasoned that the combined effects of so many different substances could in no way be known. He came rapidly to the conclusion that blood-letting, enemas and emetics weakened the already ill patients and could in no way help towards a cure, and he campaigned against such practices for most of his life. Such was his disillusionment that he gave up the practice of medicine for a while and supported himself and his growing family by undertaking translation work, at the same time pursuing his chemical and botanical studies.

It was in the course of his translation work that he received in 1790 the stimulus which led him to his radical rethink of medical treatment. While translating a treatise by the Scottish physician Dr William Cullen on the use of cinchona or Peruvian bark in the treatment of intermittent fever (malaria), he was struck by Cullen's assertion that the therapeutic effects of cinchona were due to its tonic, bitter and astringent qualities. Hahnemann disagreed with this opinion and as a result of self-experimentation with it rediscovered the forgotten principle of treatment by similars.

As he was a brilliant classical scholar, it is possible that he realized that what he had discovered was in line with one of Hippocrates' systems, formulated so many centuries before. He began experimenting with other drugs in use at the time and, using his extensive knowledge of botany, he investigated the effects of a number of medicinal plants, both on himself and on a small circle of friends and pupils. Over the next twenty years or so he established the basis of the homoeopathic materia medica.

In 1796 he published an article in which he stated that there were three ways in which to approach the treatment of disease:

● The first was to remove or destroy the cause of the illness if known – in other words, preventive medicine.

● The second was the commonly used treatment by opposites – in other words, palliative treatment such as laxatives for constipation, which he considered to be a false path.

● The third was the treatment by similars which he stated was the only sure way, apart from prevention, to treat disease.

He also stressed the importance of a sensible diet, fresh air, plenty of exercise and good hygiene as being pre-requisites of a healthy life – factors which were almost entirely ignored by or unknown to the majority of his colleagues. Homoeopathy officially came into being in 1796 (although this name did not appear in print until 1807) and the first edition of his *Organon of Rational Healing* was published in Dresden in 1810. This volume described his experiences with the similia principle and expressed his ideas about disease and its treatment. It ran to five editions in his life-time, with a sixth completed just before he died but not published until many years later.

Having discovered and developed a logical and effective system of treatment, Hahnemann returned to medical practice in 1805. He maintained that treatment should be carried out in the gentlest possible way available and that it should be both speedy and lasting. He was also of the opinion that remedies should be given singly and not in mixtures as was the custom. He was well aware that many of his remedies were extremely poisonous in crude doses and from this developed his system of serial dilution and succussion as he experimented with successive dilutions in order to achieve a healing effect without producing toxic side-effects. Although he started out using crude, undiluted tinctures, towards the end of his life he was using very high potencies.

Hahnemann's opposition to the ignorance and barbarism of the medicine of his day made him many enemies in the medical profession. He also incurred the anger of the apothecaries who were afraid of being put out of business if all their complex mixtures were swept away. Hahnemann therefore had to move frequently as restrictions on his practice were imposed in one town after another, but despite this he lectured for a time on homoeopathy in the University of Leipzig and he had a large band of influential patrons and supporters as well as a number of able and gifted pupils. For most of his career after discovering the similia principle, he was inundated with more patients than the average practitioner could have coped with. Towards the end of his long life he married for the second time. His new wife was a Parisian and he spent the last eight years of his life in Paris, where he continued to practise until he died in 1843 at the age of eighty-eight.

By that time homoeopathy had spread to all parts of Europe (except Norway and Sweden), to Britain, America, Mexico, Cuba and Russia, and shortly afterwards it reached India and South America. In 1832 Dr Frederick Foster Hervey Quinn introduced it to Britain, where, despite opposition from the orthodox practitioners, it quickly spread to various parts of the country. Hahnemann and his homoeopathy had already gained considerable prestige from his success in treating the typhus epidemic which swept into Europe in the wake of Napoleon's retreat from Moscow in 1813. Homoeopathy again proved its superiority over the orthodox methods of treatment during the great cholera epidemic which raged across Europe in 1831. The usual death rate was more than 50 per cent of those affected, but with homoeopathic treatment it was usually between 5 per cent and 16 per cent. In the London cholera epidemic of 1854, the death rate in the orthodox London hospitals was 53.2 per cent and in the London homoeopathic hospital it was 16.4 per cent – a striking difference.

It was largely this greater efficacy in the treatment of epidemic infections which were such a scourge in those days that allowed homoeopathy to spread so quickly. Its gentle approach and its emphasis on sensible preventive measures also gave it considerable patient appeal when compared with the more barbarous established approaches. It made great strides, especially in America, where Hahnemann's pupil Dr Constantine Hering finally settled. He had already discovered the therapeutic power of lachesis, the deadly poison of the Surukuku or Bushmaster snake of the Amazon forests, and his *Guiding Symptoms*, written in 1879, is still in use today. Other able practitioners of homoeopathy in America were Allen, Nash, Boenninghausen and Boericke – all of whom added to the homoeopathic literature and whose work is still used today by students of homoeopathy.

In Britain Dr Richard Hughes introduced modifications into Hahnemann's original teachings in order to popularize homoeopathy and to make it simpler to prescribe. Hughes advocated the use of low potencies prescribed on pathological grounds rather than on the patient's general symptom picture. These low potencies were often given over long periods, and frequently mixtures of different remedies were used.

In America Dr James Tyler Kent was appalled by such modifications, feeling that many of the practices which Hahnemann had campaigned against had crept into the practice of homoeopathy itself in the one hundred or so years since its rediscovery. Kent urged the use of the single remedy chosen on the totality of the patient's symptoms and not repeated as long as an improvement was maintained. He also stated that although in acute illness low potencies could be effective, in chronic conditions high potencies were much more likely to produce good results if the most similar remedy could be discerned. He gave many lectures on the materia medica which are still widely used today, and undertook a systematic classification of all the symptoms and signs produced by the remedies. This enormous work, known as Kent's *Repertory of the Homoeopathic Materia Medica*, is of great use to all homoeopathic practitioners. Boenninghausen had previously produced a repertory but it contained many more remedies under each heading than Kent's repertory, which is easier to use.

With Kent's insistence on adherence to Hahnemann's original principles, two schools of homoeopathy arose and considerable animosity developed between them. There was the high potency, single dose, classical Kentian school, and the low potency, often-repeated school of Hughes. Many practitioners these days combine both schools of thought, using repeated doses of low potencies for pathological prescribing: for example, Rhustoxicodendron 6X twice a day for a period of several weeks in cases of arthritis where the condition is aggravated by damp weather and rest; and giving, at the same time, a single dose of a high potency prescribed on constitutional grounds – that is, the whole symptom complex of the patient.

Hahnemann was ahead of his time in advocating preventive medicine, as well as in his use of homoeopathy. These effective treatments, along with his rejection of blood-letting, purging and polypharmacy which weakened rather than helped the patient, gave homoeopathy the edge over orthodox therapy for most of the nineteenth century. Patients appreciated a more understanding approach, and orthodox practitioners themselves came to realize the harm caused by their traditional practices and gradually rejected them, while at the same time adopting the sensible preventive measures. This, coupled with the decline of the great infectious epidemics which gave homoeopathy its signal successes, eliminated much of the gap between the orthodox and homoeopathic schools and eroded much of the latter's popularity. Also, Lister's discovery of the importance of antisepsis made surgery, which up till that time had been a hazardous technique, a safe procedure, and with the development of anaesthesia, surgery suddenly began to enjoy great popularity as a panacea for many ills. Finally, the discovery of replacement therapy with hormones and vitamins and the introduction of the antibiotics allowed orthodox medical treatment itself to begin to make great strides. With the increasing array of modern pharmaceuticals which have been developed in the last forty years or so, the concept of treatment with opposites has once more dwarfed the concept of treatment with similars which has never been accepted by the medical establishment.

This tremendous progress of conventional medicine in the present century has confirmed belief in the treatment by opposites. It seemed as if it would not be long before a treatment was found for every disease. The great infectious epidemics responded to a combination of improved sanitation and hygiene, vaccination programmes and antibiotics. Knowledge of vitamin and hormone deficiencies and their replacement brought new hope to sufferers from diabetes, pernicious anaemia and a host of other disorders. Cortisone was hailed as a wonder drug for a whole host of skin problems and inflammatory disorders. Optimism ran high.

But what has happened to all the bright promises? Where is the excellent health we have all come to expect? It was found that antibiotics could have side-effects. But not only that. Some acupuncturists find that they cannot treat patients who have had long courses of antibiotic therapy until several months after this treatment has finished. The antibiotics can have an adverse effect on the body's response mechanisms, possibly some aspect of the immune system. And if our defence mechanism is impaired, what other dangers may we not be open to? First it was the different forms of hepatitis virus which caused alarm. Now we have Legionnaire's Disease and AIDS. It seems as though we have conquered the traditional infectious diseases only to be assaulted by new ones.

Nearly two hundred years ago, Hahnemann considered that the treatment of chronic illness was the greatest challenge to medicine and he spent many years of his life working on this problem. The aspect of the disease statistics of the twentieth century which strikes us most is the tremendous rise, particularly since the Second World War, in the incidence of all chronic diseases, which prove more and more difficult to treat despite the vast array of modern pharmaceutical drugs now available. What can have gone wrong?

One facile explanation is that with the eradication of the infectious fevers people are living longer, and so are now living into the age groups where chronic diseases start to manifest themselves. Formerly, we are told, people died before they had much time to develop these diseases. But is this really the explanation, or could there be other factors at work?

We go back yet again to Hahnemann, who strongly advocated preventive medicine and included in this a healthy life-style. Good hygiene we now have. With our largely sedentary life-styles, however, the amount of fresh air and exercise obtained by most of us is sadly limited. But when it comes to diet, we are probably as badly off if not worse than people were in Hahnemann's day. Since the end of the last war more and more of our food has been subjected to factory processing, with the concomitant addition of more and more chemical additives to counteract the deterioration in taste, texture, colour and palatability which the processing of food brings about. This, along with the increasing use of biocides (herbicides, pesticides and fungicides) in food-crop production, and factory-farming methods of rearing livestock (with increasing reliance on antibiotics, hormones and other drugs), has reduced the quality of the food we eat and has probably rendered much of it actually harmful. The chemical stress on the body from unnecessary, unwanted and possibly toxic chemical additives is probably an important factor in the tremendous rise in chronic ill-health in this country. It is interesting that the rise in chronic disease parallels the rise in the chemicalization of our food.

However, the changes in the quality of our food are probably not the whole story. As we saw when we discussed the principles of homoeopathy, treatment by similars aims at improving the body's resistance to diseases and expects to cure from within, out. In the process of treating chronic disease, the patient often experiences a recurrence of old symptoms, and this can be distressing for a time. Treatment by opposites, on the other hand, works by palliating and suppressing symptoms. Indeed, many categories of drugs indicate this in their names – for instance, the antibiotics, antidepressants, antispasmodics, anti-inflammatories, antacids and so on. But what happens when symptoms are suppressed? Is this not working in the opposite direction to treatment by similars and driving the imbalances, the illnesses, deeper into the system? The use of topical steroid creams to treat eczema can certainly clear the skin up miraculously, but the patient may then go on to develop asthma. Asthma and eczema often alternate, the skin being worse when the asthma is better. More and more we are beginning to suspect that a similar situation may also occur with other conditions and that the suppression of symptoms with palliative therapy leads to the development, perhaps even years later, of more serious complaints. The increased expansion of the pharmaceutical industry also parallels the rise in chronic disease.

Quite apart from the side-effects of pharmaceutical drugs, which seem to be reported with increasing frequency these days, it may well turn out that such therapies have the less obvious effect of further imbalancing the body's mechanisms, so adding to the burden of chronic ill-health. Thus it may not be only the antibiotics which are associated with long-term disadvantages but the great majority of the synthetic pharmaceutical drugs upon which modern medicine relies. That these drugs themselves may actually be adding to that incidence is a disturbing thought. However, the fact that disease incidence continues to rise must surely attest to the inadequacy of such drugs to cope with it.

Perhaps the greatest number of casualties among the modern pharmaceuticals occurs in the realm of the antibiotics as one after another falls victim to the amazing abilities of bacteria to adapt to them, so that more new ones continually have to be developed. This is an area of increasing concern, since it is feared that we may well run out of useful antibiotics, which would leave us defenceless in the face of overwhelming attack by resistant organisms.

Looking back over our century one cannot help feeling that despite all the research, the new drugs and the improved surgical techniques, to say nothing of the introduction of health services in many western countries, the health of our societies has declined rather than improved. Perhaps it is time to ask ourselves whether the notion of treatment by opposites, which has held the stage for so long, is indeed the false path that Hahnemann considered it to be. Is an unbiased reappraisal of the concept of treatment by similars long overdue?

This approach to treatment, strong in the nineteenth century and all but eclipsed in the twentieth, is still waiting in the wings. Its therapies have stood the test of time and are as effective today as they were two hundred years ago. The remedies of the homoeopathic materia medica have not, as has happened to their orthodox counterparts, had to be abandoned, as one after another they have lost their efficacy or have been shown to be too toxic to be used safely. The tide is beginning to turn back to a gentler, safer and more effective approach to the treatment of ill-health and disease.

Despite the decline in its popularity, homoeopathy has not been standing still for the entire twentieth century. A number of remedies have been added to the materia medica including the bowel nosodes which were first discovered by Dr Edward Bach and later added to by Dr John Paterson. These nosodes (remedies prepared from abnormal bowel flora) are in the same category as other nosodes such as variolinum, morbillinum, pertussin and diphtherinum which are prepared from smallpox, measles, whooping cough and diphtheria respectively. A nosode remedy can be prepared from any infectious disease and used, in a manner similar to isopathy, to counteract the effects of that disease. This aspect of homoeopathy is the one most akin to the vaccinations of the orthodox approach which are really a homoeopathic application.

Hahnemann and his followers left us a legacy of many hundreds of remedies and the number has continued to grow until at the present time there are between two and three thousand remedies in the homoeopathic materia medica, each with its remedy picture, some of which have been more extensively worked out than others.

It is therefore a problem for the homoeopathic practitioner to learn these pictures, many of which are somewhat similar, sufficiently well to be able to match accurately each patient with the correct remedy. This is particularly a problem in chronic disease. An approach to simplifying this task was first made by Boenninghausen and later by Kent when they produced their repertories, or collections of symptoms and signs common to each remedy. The idea was to obtain as many outstanding characteristics as possible from the patient and then to find the remedy, or remedies, which contained them all. In recent years this idea has been computerized to aid in remedy selection and several computer programs now exist.

Another approach to the problem of chronic prescribing is that which has been developed by Vithoulkas in Greece, Orthega in Mexico, and Masi and Paschero in Argentina – that of finding the essence of the remedies, or the scarlet thread or idea running through all the various aspects of the remedy picture. This essence or idea, which is based on a psychological evaluation, is then matched with the essence of the patient in question. Orthega and Paschero, however, consider all diseases to be due to environmental causes and miss out on the inherited factors present in the cause of the disease. Both Paschero and Masi think that disorders in the spiritual sphere underlie all chronic conditions, but while Orthega argues that several different remedies may have to be used before the patient can be cured, treating each layer as it presents rather like peeling an onion, both Paschero and Masi advocate just *one* remedy for each patient and consider that the patient does not change the chronic remedy at all throughout life.

This is not the experience of the majority of prescribers, however, and approaches such as psionic medicine and bio-electronic regulatory medicine find that a number of different remedies are always indicated in a chronic case. These two recent developments will be dealt with more fully in the final chapter.

It is therefore obvious that different approaches to the problem of chronic disease exist and that much research will be required before the position can be clarified. None of the more recent views invalidates Hahnemann's original discoveries or teachings, and the approach in Europe, including Vithoulkas's school, continues to be largely Hahnemannian.

CHAPTER SEVEN

HOW DOES

HOMOEOPATHY

WORK?

By their very nature both this chapter which deals with current ideas on how homoeopathy works and Chapter 9 which reviews some of the evidence that it does work are inevitably somewhat scientific and technical. If you, the reader, are not of a scientific bent, then they may not much appeal to you and you may wish to gloss over them. They are intended for those who like to probe into the whys and wherefores of things or who like to assess fully the credentials of a subject before they give it serious consideration. The omission of these chapters will not detract from your general appreciation of homoeopathy.

In potencies higher than the 12C the chances of even a single molecule of the original starting material still being present become more and more remote. This fact, quite unknown when Hahnemann first discovered the effects of potentization, has been a major stumbling block to the acceptance of homoeopathy by orthodox doctors. If none of the original material is left in the preparation, how can it possibly have any therapeutic effect?

Since its discovery by Avogadro in the early part of the nineteenth century, this knowledge has also become a major problem for homoeopathic practitioners. By the simple laws of dilution, solutions beyond the 12C potency should have no activity whatsoever, and yet clinically they can be shown to have an effect and, what is more, higher potencies often show more powerful effects than lower potencies. How is this possible?

We do not yet know what it is in a homoeopathic potency that has a curative action, nor do we know how homoeopathic remedies work in the body any more than we know the mechanisms of action of many of the conventional drugs used in medicine. Where drug actions are known, they have been found to exert an effect on the body's metabolic processes – that is, our inner chemical workings – inhibiting or stimulating enzyme function or having an effect on their control mechanisms. There is therefore no reason to suppose that the homoeopathic remedies are any different. If they are going to affect the body's functioning, they also must act through the biochemical, metabolic level.

Much of this chapter is hypothesis, but hypothesis based on known facts. It attempts to draw together information from several different fields and to construct from this information a theory of how homoeopathic remedies may work. The ideas expressed may well be wide of the mark, or they may not be, but this does not really matter since the purpose of hypotheses is to stimulate more ideas, and the research to either confirm or refute them. If they achieve this then they are of value, irrespective of whether they, themselves, are right or wrong.

To get some idea of a possible solution to the problem that in potencies higher than the 12C none of the original starting material is likely to remain in the potency, we have to go back to some basic concepts of chemistry. Chemical reactions and the compounds which they form all depend, ultimately, on the way the electrons are arranged in the individual atoms involved; the reactions being such as to achieve a stable configuration of electrons in the orbits of each participating atom (see Figure 4, p.55). The electrons are one type of sub-atomic particle mentioned in Chapter 4.

They are also what constitutes electricity. Molecules thus take up a specific shape, and this shape is particularly important in the complex organic molecules formed by living systems. Stereospecificity, or shape-specificity, is the hallmark of biochemistry and even small changes in the shapes of molecules can have profound effects throughout the body.

For example, the genetic material is made up from a complex molecule known as DNA (deoxyribonucleic acid). This itself is built up from long chains of sugar and phosphate molecules to which are attached nitrogen-containing molecules called the nucleotide bases. There are four possible bases, and specific arrangements of these form the genes which transmit the inherited characteristics from one generation to another. All the complex information which is passed on from one generation to the next is coded using specific arrangements of just four molecules!

The genes code information for the formation of protein, the main constituent of our tissues and enzymes. Just one base wrong in a particular DNA sequence may cause a coding error in the protein formed by that gene. An example of a condition caused in this way is phenylketonuria – one of the so-called 'inborn errors of metabolism' – an inherited biochemical disorder for which babies are now routinely tested within a few days of birth. In this condition, one wrong base pair in the DNA of the gene coding for a particular enzyme means that this enzyme is functionless and the body cannot easily make melanin, which is the dark pigment responsible for brown eyes and dark hair, and which is produced in response to sunlight when we get a sun-tan. This, therefore, results in a child who tends to be fair-haired and blue-eyed. This in itself would be no drawback. The serious symptom of phenylketonuria is the development of mental retardation, sometimes accompanied by convulsions, which results from toxic products formed by the body's attempt to bypass the block. All this results from just one mistake in a shape-specific complex molecule. The treatment, in the case of phenylketonuria, is to put the baby on to a phenylalanine-free diet, thus bypassing the metabolic block, and this is why it is important to diagnose the condition as soon after birth as possible. This is just one example of the many that could be quoted to emphasize the importance of shape in biological systems.

Energy storage is also shape-specific. Living systems store their energy in the cells as specific high-energy phosphate bonds linked to molecules similar to those used to build up the genes.

Homoeopathic potencies are diluted in water/alcohol mixtures – the water being the solvent (the substance which does the dissolving) and the alcohol being present as a preservative. Now water is a most anomalous liquid with many strange and unexpected characteristics.[1] It is the only substance, liquid at normal temperatures, which expands when it solidifies or freezes – a property shared only by diamond, silicon and germanium, three solids whose structures are related to that of ice. All other materials contract when they solidify. In addition water can form several different kinds of crystals. If it is frozen at different atmospheric pressures, the ice crystals formed are different. The high-pressure ices have specific crystal patterns which differ with the pressure used to form them, and which also differ from the patterns of ice formed at normal atmospheric pressure. In fact water can form at least nine different types of ice crystal. Water also has a melting point and a boiling point much higher than would be expected from its formula and it becomes more fluid with increasing temperature. In fact, from its formula one would expect it to be a gas at normal temperatures but it is a liquid. These anomalous properties of water may turn out to be of

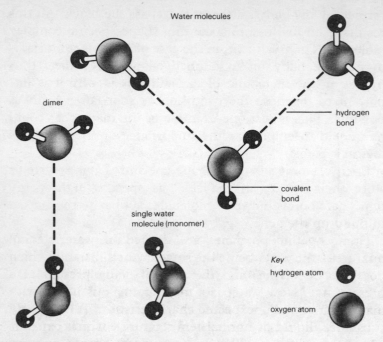

Water molecules

dimer

hydrogen
bond

covalent
bond

single water
molecule (monomer)

Key
hydrogen atom

oxygen atom

Figure 7. Water molecules

considerable importance in the preparation of homoeopathic remedies.

Current ideas of the structure of water visualize it as being composed of a random network of molecules linked together by hydrogen bonds (Figure 7),[2,3] some of which are strained or even broken, but with a general structure not unlike that which is found in ordinary ice, also known as hexagonal ice to distinguish it from its variant form, cubic ice, which is formed at lower temperatures. These are both ices formed at normal atmospheric pressure.

In hexagonal ice the water molecules are arranged in such a way that they form an open lattice structure which produces puckered layers of hydrogen-bonded water molecules (Figure 8). This type of structure is a very inefficient

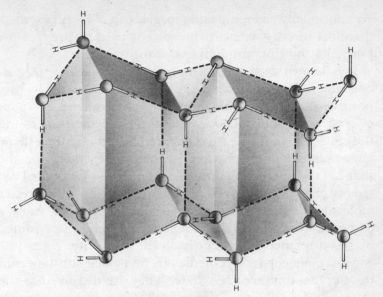

Figure 8. The structure of hexagonal ice

way of filling space because it contains a regular network of empty spaces which run both parallel to, and at right angles to, the puckered lattice layers. It is this open structure which makes ice less dense than water, and accounts for the fact that it floats.[4]

When ice melts it is believed that this structure is largely maintained but that the spaces become partly filled, possibly by unbonded water molecules which are small enough to fit inside them, or are reduced in size by bending and reorganization of the hydrogen bonds. As the water gets warmer, it is visualized that the structure becomes more random, thus accounting for the increased fluidity of the water at higher temperatures.

Water is therefore no longer seen as a simple collection of individual water molecules, but as a complex random network of molecules linked together by hydrogen bonds and forming extensive three-dimensional structures which are continually changing and reorganizing. Water polymers therefore already exist in the solvent used to prepare the potencies, but in a random and disordered form.

It is known that when a non-polar substance – that is, one which does not ionize like salts, acids and alkalis into positive and negative components – is dissolved in water, or a water/alcohol mixture, the water polymers surround the molecules of the dissolved material, and take up a shape known as the solvation cage,[1] which is dependent on the shape of the starting material, but which also gives the least strain on the hydrogen bonds connecting the water molecules (Figure 9). The water polymers thus have a pattern imposed upon them, a pattern which is determined by the substance which is dissolved, the solute.

Most homoeopathic remedies are non-polar substances in their crude, unpotentized state. They are dissolved in the water/alcohol solvent. Energy is then put into the system by the process of succussion and it is visualized that this energy input helps to stabilize the shape-specific water polymers so formed. As more energy is put in at each dilution stage, the water polymer chains become longer and longer, and presumably at some stage break, forming a number of shorter lengths of water polymer. As the original solute is successively diluted, so the mirroring, shape-specific water polymers build up and continue to pass on the shape-encoded information to successive potencies long after the original starting material has been diluted out. The information inherent in the crude remedy is thus transmitted to the diluting fluid by means of the energy contained in the succussion process. The situation is analogous to the way in which the genes with their shape-specificity pass on inherited characteristics from one generation to the next. The relationship between the homoeopathic potency and the original starting material may be similar to the relationship between an antigen and

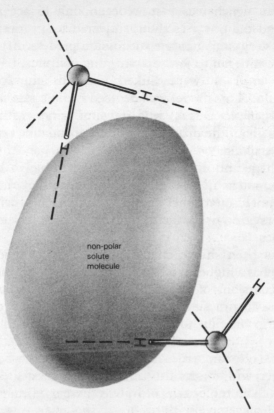

non-polar
solute
molecule

Figure 9. Water molecules surrounding the solute to form a solvation cage

its specific antibody. They are both complementary shape-specific molecular systems.

In this connection it is appropriate to mention a model which was demonstrated at a genetics meeting in London some years ago. This model consisted of a number of wooden blocks which represented isolated sections of the genetic material, the DNA, and each had intricate hinged sections at either end. Each block appeared to be complete in itself and all were identical. The blocks were placed in a long tray which was just wide enough to accommodate them and the tray was then subjected to a series of sharp shocks, very similar to the succussion process. After a time, the blocks began to join up, forming couplets, triplets and so on, until all were linked to form one long-chain 'molecule'. This model was devised to illustrate properties of the genetic DNA, but its similarities with current theories about the production of homoeopathic remedies is indeed striking.

As shape and energy are interchangeable in biological systems, and as all biological reactions are shape-specific, it is not unreasonable to suggest that shape-specific water polymers are the basis of the activity of homoeopathic potencies.

It has been shown that a potency of a homoeopathic remedy has a higher viscosity than a straight dilution, without succussion, of the same remedy repeated the same number of times, suggesting that large molecules are present in the potency which do not occur in the straight dilution.[5] Infra-red spectroscopic studies[6] and nuclear magnetic resonance measurements[7] of potentized solutions compared with straight dilutions also suggest the presence of long-chain molecules, although these studies have yet to be confirmed.

In this connection it is interesting that high temperatures, strong sunlight and certain types of radiation destroy homoeopathic potencies, and that these are agents which are known to destroy long-chain polymers. Consider, for instance, the effects of heat and sunlight on plastics which are also long-chain polymers.

Modern theories of water structure centre on computer-simulation models from which has been developed a concept which is similar to the DNA model just discussed, the concept of cellular automata.[8] A cellular automaton is a mathematical model which has, like DNA, the power of self-replication, and the principle of cellular automata is believed to underlie a number of the phenomena seen in the natural world, such as the complex patterns of colour on the shells of some molluscs, the coat patterns of some mammalian species and the vortex patterns of water. As applied to water, they are visualized as being particular polywater formations which have the power to impress their pattern on the surrounding water polymers. The presence, in a volume of water, of even one such cellular automaton would be enough to impress the pattern on the whole of that body of water. The homoeopathic potencies, being structured water polymers, can be visualized as being more powerful than the random water polymers present in the body fluids. They can therefore be visualized as potential cellular automata capable of imprinting their pattern on the surrounding body fluids. It is similar to reprogramming a computer, with the remedies being the program. If this is indeed the case, it would explain why a small dose of a remedy can effect a major change in the clinical condition of patients.

At the biochemical level the homoeopathic remedies are believed, by some practitioners at least, to key into metabolic cycles — that is, the body's basic biochemical reactions.

The body is in a continual state of chemical activity. The food we eat is broken down by means of a series of enzymes in the mouth, stomach and small intestine to its simple component molecules which can then be absorbed into the bloodstream. Once inside the body these simple molecules are used to repair damaged or worn out cell components, to form energy storage compounds or to provide immediate energy to power the cells, tissues and the body as a whole. These transformations are accomplished by means of stepwise reactions, each of which is mediated by a specific enzyme. The enzymes are specialized proteins which enable the body to carry out at body heat and atmospheric pressure complex reactions which, if man were able to reproduce them at all, would require high temperatures and high pressures to accomplish. The enzymes are therefore essential to the body's proper and harmonious functioning. Blocks in enzyme function, due either to deficiency or absence of an enzyme (as in phenylketonuria), can cause severe disruption of the body's metabolic pathways. Even small degrees of enzyme inefficiency can have effects on other pathways if these are dependent for their functioning on products of the defective pathway or if they are inhibited by the build-up of substances prior to the block.

We are learning more and more about the body's complex system of integrated metabolic pathways – for instance, the recent discovery of the prostaglandin system – but much, much more remains to be discovered.

The various components of the prostaglandin system occur fleetingly, and in minute amounts, in all the tissues of the body. This system has links with many other aspects of the body's metabolism, from the hormonal system to the immune system, tissue repair and the transport of substances across cell membranes. In fact it may well turn out that components of the prostaglandin system are involved in all aspects of the integration and harmonization of body processes.

An example of the far-reaching effects of defects in prostaglandin synthesis or control is the disease known as systemic lupus erythematosis, S L E. This is one of the so-called auto-immune group of diseases in which the body produces antibodies to its own tissues, and thus begins to destroy them. The symptoms of this condition include fever and inflammatory changes in the connective or fibrous tissues of the body, increased fibrous tissue production, baldness, sensitivity to sunlight, kidney failure, high blood pressure, heart involvement, an increased risk of

abortion, defects in the immune system, psychotic manifestations and neurological problems similar to multiple
sclerosis. It can involve almost any system of the body and
yet there is evidence that it could be the result of a single
gene defect, or defects in a limited number of genes. There
is considerable evidence[9] that the multitudinous aspects of
S L E may be the result of deficiencies of two members of the
prostaglandin group of substances and excesses of others,
which could be the result either of one or two related defects
in the prostaglandin pathway, or of a single basic defect.

Such wide-reaching results are remarkably reminiscent
of the drug pictures of many of the homoeopathic remedies,
which are visualized as being the keys which can unlock
various metabolic blocks. If such varied symptoms can be
the result of a single defect, or of one or two related defects,
it is quite conceivable that a homoeopathic remedy, acting
to eliminate the block, can have equally far-reaching effects.
This, of course, has been observed in practice. Since there
are many hundreds, if not thousands, of enzymes in the
body, the number of potential metabolic blocks is indeed
large – large enough to accommodate all the remedies of
the homoeopathic materia medica. Indeed, the results of
recent research suggest that abnormalities of prostaglandin
metabolism may lie at the heart of the majority of the
chronic degenerative diseases – defects in particular
enzymes giving rise to different aspects of chronic disease.
Studies of homoeopathic remedies in relation to prostaglandin metabolism may therefore yield interesting and
fruitful results.

The remedies of the homoeopathic materia medica are
derived from all the kingdoms of nature – the mineral,
plant and animal realms. The cells and tissues of all living
creatures, including ourselves, depend on a number of
mineral elements and radicals – in particular, sodium,
potassium, calcium, magnesium, manganese, copper, iron,

cobalt, zinc, phosphate, sulphate and chloride – for their proper functioning. Without them, indeed, we could not live. In fact, it is likely that all the elements which exist in the earth's crust are present, albeit in infinitesimal amounts, in our bodies.

In an earlier chapter we described a few of the complex relationships which exist between different species and different kingdoms of nature. Individual behaviour, particularly in the insect world, is now known to be regulated by means of molecules known as pheromones, which are possibly analogous to our prostaglandins and hormones. These molecules are air-borne and present in only trace amounts, but they control the behaviour of particular species of insects over remarkably long distances.

Many basic metabolic pathways show striking similarities throughout the bacterial, plant and animal kingdoms. The more basic and important to life a particular metabolic process is, the less likely is it to have changed significantly throughout evolution. For instance, the basic genetic material is similar. The more highly evolved forms have more genes controlling more processes, but even viral and bacterial genetic material is similar to some parts of our own. Haemoglobin, the oxygen-carrying pigment in our blood, shows small species variations, but is basically similar all the way from fish to man. Its analogue in the plant world is chlorophyll, which catalyses the splitting of the water molecule and the production of oxygen. Chlorophyll, interestingly, is similar to vitamin B_{12} which is essential, along with other vitamins and minerals, for the proper functioning of our haemoglobin-carrying cells, the red cells of the blood. The process of glycolysis, the first stage in the utilization of glucose to produce energy, is similar in bacteria and in our own muscles. Many substances of vegetable origin have profound pharmacological effects on animal cells and tissues.

It would seem that nature is remarkably economical, despite the apparent diversity of natural forms. Just as all the genetic information that can be conceived of is coded for by just four molecules, and all the proteins that exist are built up from just twenty amino acids, so efficient biochemical systems once established tend to be preserved. Metabolic similarities and correspondences therefore exist throughout all life. Homoeopathy, with its remedies drawn from the mineral, plant and animal kingdoms, may well hold within its materia medica the stereospecific, or shape-specific, keys to unlock many of the blocks which can occur in our internal functioning – our metabolic processes.

Metabolic blocks can occur for a variety of reasons:

● First, there can be defects in an enzyme, either in its amount or in its function, causing either a partial or total block at a specific point in a metabolic pathway.

● Second, blocks may be caused by a deficiency of enzyme co-factors – that is, various vitamin or trace element deficiencies.

● Third, blocks may be caused by toxic substances inhibiting the function of an enzyme or enzymes.

● Fourth (less obviously), there are blocks caused by bacterial or viral toxins or byproducts which affect cellular function, or blocks caused by the insertion of viral DNA into our own genome, our own genetic material.

● Fifth, structural blocks can occur caused by injuries, scar tissue and so on.

● Sixth, there are blocks caused by emotional upsets possibly affecting hormone function – for example, adrenaline which is released in fright situations.

● Seventh, there may be blocks to the flow of electrical energy in the acupuncture meridians.

● Finally, on a more subtle level, there may be mental blocks which can have an effect on the emotional and physical planes. The concepts of mind over matter to overcome problems, and the reverse process where fear of an illness can produce that illness, illustrate the part such mental factors can play.

Most of the blocks mentioned here are at the physical level, but the emotional and mental blocks are equally important. As we saw in a previous chapter, all the planes or levels of the human being interact with one another, and defects arising in one can be experienced by the others and can cause upsets in them. An analogous situation is where a stone is dropped into a pond. The ripples spread out from the point where the stone is dropped and can affect a great area of the pond and perhaps even the whole of it. The imbalance thus spreads out from the initial focus or storm centre. The homoeopathic remedies with their powerful patterning effect, perhaps along the lines of cellular automata concepts, are visualized as spreading through the body and counteracting the imbalance, so restoring the tissues to harmony and balance.

This concept of homoeopathic drug action can be used to estimate how often, in theory at least, a remedy may have to be repeated – an aspect of homoeopathic prescribing which causes great difficulty and debate.

If the disturbance was the result of a single adverse stimulus, such as a sudden fright, a bereavement or an infection, which is now no longer operating although its effects persist, then theoretically one dose of the appropriate remedy should be sufficient to re-pattern the system and set things to rights. If, however, the stimulus is a recurring one, then presumably one dose of the remedy would not necessarily be sufficient to hold the system in balance, as repeated assaults are being experienced. Repetitions of the remedy would therefore be required.

It can be postulated that the programming effect of high potencies is greater than that of low potencies. Therefore, if a low potency is being used, it may be necessary to administer repeated doses to achieve the same effect as a single dose of a higher potency. In practice, low potencies are usually prescribed over a period of time, whereas high potencies are classically administered as the single dose. The exception to this is the acute situation where high potencies are repeated at rapid intervals. The acute situation, however, can be visualized as being one in which repeated assaults are being inflicted, requiring repeated administration of the appropriate remedy to re-balance the system. Repetition of the remedy is continued for as long as is required, and the doses are tailed off gradually.

It has been suggested by Dennis Milner – doctor of science in the metallurgy department at Birmingham University who has carried out much research into etheric force-field photography – that the different potency levels relate to the different planes of being in the following way:

- low potencies up to 12C (physical plane)

- intermediate potencies, 30C, 200C (emotional plane)

- high potencies, M, 10M, 50M, CM and higher (mental plane).

This concept is in keeping with the observations from the remedy provings, since the low potencies produce mainly physical symptoms, and the high potencies are required to bring out the full mental symptomatology.

In the early days of homoeopathy, Hahnemann's most striking successes were with the epidemic diseases – cholera, typhus, typhoid and the like. Acute conditions usually resolved successfully under homoeopathic treatment. However Hahnemann came increasingly to recognize that there were patients whose diseases continually seemed to relapse, or change their form, and such patients could be extremely difficult to treat. These were people suffering from chronic diseases.

After much study Hahnemann came to the conclusion that the basic underlying causes of chronic diseases were what he termed the inherited miasms,[10] a term which we might translate into modern parlance as inherited predispositions. He described three miasms (syphilis, sycosis and psora) which he related to the venereal diseases (syphilis and gonorrhoea) and the skin itch (akin to psoriasis) respectively. Nowadays the list of miasms has been extended to include the tubercular miasms, measles, whooping cough, vaccinia, diphtheria and so on. Miasms are now recognized to be both inherited and acquired; and often a specific remedy called a nosode, which is related to the infection in question, is required before a chronic condition can be entirely cleared up.

Hahnemann's theory of miasms attracted a great deal of scorn and scepticism in his day, and this attitude has tended to persist, particularly in orthodox medical circles. However it would appear that Hahnemann was a couple of centuries ahead of his time because it is now known that the DNA of certain viruses can incorporate itself into our own genome, our own inherited material. If this happens in a germ cell, it has the chance of being passed on to future generations. If even one base pair change in DNA can profoundly affect the body, the inclusion of a whole length of foreign genetic material among our own genes could easily give rise to metabolic imbalances and disturbances.

So perhaps Hahnemann was quite right when he suggested that inherited factors from past infections or infections suffered by ancestors caused imbalances which lay at the heart of the chronic diseases. Not only may viruses incorporate themselves into our DNA, but there is now a suggestion that some viruses at least may have arisen from bits of our own DNA which have escaped from our cells and become so modified as to be capable of independent existence.

Advances in molecular biology in recent years have served to emphasize the possible relationships between homoeopathy, immunology and genetics. All are profoundly dependent on shape-specificity for their functioning.

Hahnemann's conception of disease being due to a combination of intrinsic (inherited) and extrinsic (environmental) factors has turned out to be largely correct. There are a large number of rare metabolic errors which are purely hereditary and account, despite their large number, for only a small percentage of total illness, and a few conditions such as fatal poisonings which are purely environmental, but in the great majority of conditions both inherited and environmental factors are involved. Even accidents are not necessarily purely environmental since 'accident-proneness' can have inherited components, and any accident involves the mental and emotional state of the victim at the time of the accident or just prior to it (state of alertness, for instance), as well as the occurrence itself.

With homoeopathy we aim to treat the intrinsic, inherited components of the disease causation – in other words, to improve the inner state of the individual. Depending on how deep within the patient the basic disorder lies, such treatment can be anything from relatively simple to extremely complicated.

Hahnemann's first approach to the treatment of disease (Chapter 6), that of preventive medicine, aims at removing the extrinsic, environmental components. The remedies are designed to influence the internal, inherited predisposition components. A combination of these two aspects of treatment would thus appear to offer the most logical, sensible and widely applicable approach to the treatment of disease. This theme will be developed further in the next chapter.

CHAPTER EIGHT

THE RELATIONSHIP

OF HOMOEOPATHY

TO OTHER THERAPIES

The so-called 'alternative' or 'complementary' medical scene embraces a large number of different ideas, theories and treatments, many of which appear to be in conflict with each other. Patients naturally become confused by the wide number of choices available and quite rightly question the relative merits and efficacies of each.

One thing which all these therapies have in common is their belief in the innate healing powers of the body (the *vis medicatrix naturae* or healing force of nature) and they are designed to try and help the body in its natural drive to heal itself. Such therapies include homoeopathy, the Bach remedies, herbalism, acupuncture, diet therapy and naturopathy, magnetic field therapy, neural therapy, hypnotherapy and relaxation therapy, psychotherapy (including transactional analysis), cranial osteopathy, the Alexander technique, rolfing and cervical reintegration. This list is by no means exhaustive but broadly covers the field. It can be divided into five main categories:

- diet-based therapies
- postural and related therapies
- drug and remedy therapies
- electro-magnetic and related therapies
- ego-strengthening therapies aimed at treating the emotional/mental/spiritual aspects without using drugs.

It will help to understand the relationships if we consider again the diagram of the four-fold human being with its physical, emotional, mental and spiritual planes; imbalances in these planes constituting the internal or inherited factors; and the whole surrounded by environmental influences, both beneficial and harmful (Figure 10). The harmful environmental factors constitute the external factors in the production of disease (its aetiology). Disease treatment can be aimed at one or other or both of these factors.

External factors include pollution of the environment – the air, water, soil and food; infectious agents such as bacteria, viruses and other parasites; the sort of work we do, which can give rise to postural problems; the people we work and live with; the amount of exercise we take; the amount of fresh air we breathe; the amount of rest, relaxation and sleep we get, and so on.

Both the external and the internal factors can affect us at the physical, emotional, mental and spiritual levels.

1. Diet-based therapies

Taking purely environmental factors first, we can see that diet is of great importance in both the maintenance of health and in the production of disease. Basically, our diet supplies us with two things: energy to fuel ourselves, and the building blocks required to create and to replace worn out and lost components of our bodies.

Energy is measured in calories and comes principally from carbohydrates and fats, and to a lesser extent from protein. Protein is important as the source of the raw materials for building up and repairing our body tissues and our enzymes, which are largely protein. Other important ingredients which we require to keep us functioning

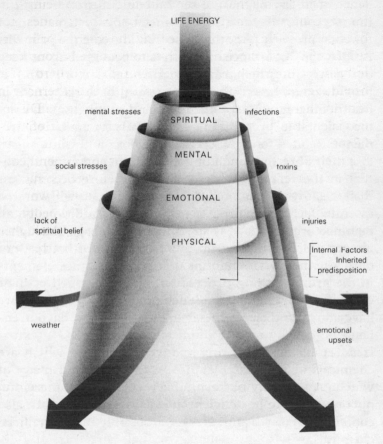

Figure 10. The interaction of the energy fields and the environment

are the vitamins, most of which are essential components of enzymes (the enzyme co-factors),[1] and minerals and trace metals, some of which are structural, such as calcium for bones and teeth, but many of which are vital components of enzyme systems or are essential for the maintenance of the electrical charges on cell membranes. If our diet is deficient in any of these essential constituents, we will in time become ill because our metabolic systems cannot function properly. Another essential ingredient of our diet is fibre, the importance of which is to provide bulk to keep our gastro-intestinal tracts working satisfactorily and to provide nourishment for the beneficial bacteria which, in health, inhabit our large intestines and supply us with a not inconsiderable proportion of our daily vitamin requirements. Refined foods, such as white flour and white sugar, lose their fibre and much of their vitamin and mineral content in the refining process. They therefore become less than healthy for us, simply empty calories without the essential factors required to utilize them. Additionally, all manufactured foods – that is, foods which go through a factory process and end up in a packet, tin or bottle – not only lose their vital vitamins, minerals and trace elements in the manufacturing process but also lose much of their colour, flavour and texture. Such processed foods therefore have added to them artificial colours, flavours, flavour enhancers (usually monosodium glutamate, MSG), texturizers, emulsifiers and preservatives – most of which are chemicals of no particular use to the body and many of which may actually be harmful. Processed food, therefore, not only tends to be deficient in essential nutrients but also contains an increasing array of possibly toxic artificial chemicals.

The chemicalization of our food extends even further than this. Increasing amounts of pesticides, herbicides and fungicides are used in agriculture and these chemicals tend to build up in the soil and are absorbed by our food plants. Since these substances are specially designed to kill life, their presence in our food is hardly beneficial.

One other less than healthy practice in connection with our diet is the fluoridation of public water supplies.

Fluoride is a powerful enzyme poison, inhibiting a number of vital enzymes in the body and causing considerable stress to our immune systems – the first line of defence against infections and other harmful environmental agents. Contrary to the official establishment line on fluoride, this substance has never been shown to be essential for body function, and its role in protecting teeth from dental caries is extremely doubtful.[2] What can be said about fluoride is that at concentrations of even less than one part per million (the official dose) it can cause toxic reactions in sensitive people and recent reassessments of the fluoridation scene suggest that this measure may be much more harmful to health than has been hitherto realized.[3] The symptoms produced by fluoride poisoning are similar to those produced by herbicides and pesticides in our food, particularly wheat. Since fluorides occur in super-phosphate fertilizers, increasing use of these in agriculture leads to increasing absorption by plants. This may be another reason for the adverse effects on some people of foods grown by current commercial agricultural methods.

This background provides the rationale of naturopathy, or nature cure, and other sensible, healthy dietary regimes. The message is to eat wholesome, fresh, unprocessed food, organically produced where possible. It is also sensible to eat foods of vegetable origin in preference to those of animal origin, to use vegetable oils rather than animal fats, and to use natural, cold-pressed vegetable oils rather than the commercially produced, processed oils.

There are a number of reasons for this advice. In the first place, today animals are often intensively reared, housed indoors under what are, for them, highly unnatural conditions. They are fed artificial diets, and to counteract the spread of infection caused by overcrowding, they require courses of antibiotics. To offset the emotional effects of their unnatural life-style they often require tranquillizers, and to ensure commercially satisfactory levels of meat production they are injected with anabolic – that is, body-building – steroid hormones. They have thus become the animal equivalents of the plants which are force-fed with artificial fertilizers and sprayed with herbicides and pesticides.

If you wish to eat animal products, then the advice is always to buy free-range produce, and to request it if it is not sold in your area. Free-range eggs and poultry are becoming more readily available. Lamb is preferable to beef and pork, as it is less likely to have been intensively reared, and game is preferable to all domestically produced meat, as it has lived under natural conditions. In general, fish is usually preferable to meat.

Animal fats tend to be saturated, whereas vegetable oils are unsaturated.[4] Fish oils are less saturated than animal fats. Domestic meat animals, and particularly those which have been intensively reared, have a considerable quantity of invisible fat in their meat whereas naturally reared animals, such as game, contain very little invisible fat.

Fats in the diet are important for two reasons. On the one hand, they are a concentrated source of energy. On the other hand, they supply us with essential fatty acids, often known as vitamin F, which are the starting materials for prostaglandin synthesis. The essential fatty acids, or E F As for short, are all polyunsaturated fatty acids, also known as P U F As. While all essential fatty acids are polyunsaturated, not all polyunsaturated fatty acids are essential. Polyunsaturated fatty acids exist in the two forms, cis and trans. The cis form is favoured by nature – another example of stereospecificity. The essential fatty acids therefore are cis form, polyunsaturated fatty acids.

Such fatty acids, however, tend to be unstable, as they are readily metabolized. They therefore have a shorter shelf-life than the trans forms and tend to turn rancid more easily. For this reason in the processing of vegetable oils, both in the extraction process and in the production of items such as margarine, food manufacturers like to convert as much of the cis fatty acid component as possible to the trans form. Unfortunately, as far as the body is concerned the trans form is valueless, apart from providing energy, and falls into the same category as saturated fat. The traditional cold-pressing method of extracting vegetable oils preserves the cis fatty acids in their natural form and therefore makes cold-pressed oils preferable to their commercially produced equivalents.

The increasing processing and chemicalization of our food and drink appears to have been a major factor in the rise of chronic disease in this country in the past three to four decades by causing much chemical stress on the body and its inner metabolic balances. Simply removing this stress can, in many instances, restore an individual to normal function without any other therapy being required. Attention to diet should therefore be a first consideration in any treatment plan to clear out toxic accumulations and correct any vitamin, mineral, trace element or fibre deficiencies.

2. Postural and related therapies

These include osteopathy, cranial osteopathy, the Alexander technique, rolfing and cervical reintegration. It was F. Matthias Alexander[5] who first stressed the importance of the cervical (neck) area in body coordination and emphasized the necessity for a correct head–neck–body relationship.

In our civilization at present, many of us have sedentary or semi-sedentary occupations. We therefore tend to be deficient in exercise and our muscles tend to become soft and flabby, and unable to keep us correctly positioned. Many of us spend much of our working day slouched over office desks, typewriters, computers or other instruments, and our leisure time slumped in front of a television set, while the journey from home to work is usually by some sort of mechanized transport – often in cars which do little to improve our posture. Small wonder that most of us have a bad posture, with much neck tension and resulting headaches, sore backs and other musculo-skeletal problems.

The therapies in this section are aimed at correcting postural deformities and reducing, or completely relieving, neck and other muscle tensions, thus allowing the body to move and function more freely. The Alexander technique achieves this slowly. Cervical reintegration is a faster method whereby pressure is exerted on muscles in tension, thus causing them to relax. The elimination of neck tension can relieve headaches, frozen shoulder, tennis elbow, wrist pain, shoulder-blade, mid-back and low-back pains, hip, knee, ankle and foot pains, lumbago, sciatica and general 'neuralgic' aches and pains, often without any other treatment being required. If a condition is simply due to muscle tension, either as a result of an injury (whiplash injury to the neck is a common one) or due to postural defects, then this type of therapy is the treatment of choice.

It is important to bear in mind, however, that muscle tension can be the result of more than just bad posture or wrong use of the body. The terms 'stiff-necked', 'tight-lipped', 'pain in the neck' and so on are part of common everyday usage, and indicate something rather deeper than a simple muscle tension problem. Such postures are often a pointer to some deeply suppressed emotion or past traumatic episode. Occasionally when using cervical reintegration to treat patients they may start to cry, or even feel faint or sick, and afterwards experience a sense of relief. Sometimes, although not always, they may remember what the suppressed or forgotten incident was.

An interesting example is the case of a man in his mid-thirties who suffered from bad neck tension and who, while having his neck treated, began to rub his hands round the sides of his chest. He then fainted for a few seconds. The treatment was discontinued but about five minutes later he suddenly remembered the reason for his unusual reaction. As a child he had played a game with some of his friends where one child would stand behind another and put his hands round the other's chest. The child in front would then take a deep breath and the one behind would tighten his arms on his chest, causing him to faint. This ploy had been completely forgotten by the patient until released along with the tension in the neck muscles by the cervical reintegration. The patient was also quite unaware that he had been rubbing his chest just prior to fainting. This is a relatively minor example of the way in which memories of past events can be locked into muscles in spasm, a subject which will be dealt with more fully in the section on ego-strengthening. It is a possibility which should always be borne in mind when neck spasm is being treated, particularly if it does not respond as expected to tension-release techniques.

Exercise is another subject which should also be considered. We all know that exercise is important for keeping our muscles in good working order. If we do not use them they tend to degenerate, a process known medically as disuse atrophy. Not only our skeletal muscles but the heart muscle also tends to degenerate if we do not get sufficient exercise, and this can lead eventually to heart failure. A certain amount of daily exercise is essential to maintain proper body tone and function, but if you are quite unused to exercise it is necessary to build up the exercise levels gradually to allow the body to acclimatize to the increased level of activity and the increased demands made on the heart and lungs, the respiratory and skeletal muscles.

There is another, more subtle effect of exercise which is to be gained from pushing ourselves periodically to the limits of our endurance, and beyond. Few of us in our modern life-styles experience this, and the nearest many of us get to exercise is the short, puffed run to catch a train or bus. When we do, however, subject ourselves to prolonged exercise, such as jogging, marathon running or mountain climbing, we experience benefits over and above the merely improved function of our hearts and musculature – benefits at the emotional, mental or spiritual levels. There is a certain satisfaction to be gained from achieving something which we thought was probably impossible for us. Somehow we break through the barrier of mental blocks with which we tend to limit ourselves and find a greater freedom of both performance and attitude. It gives us the confidence to cope with other apparently insurmountable problems, knowing that we have excelled ourselves before.

3. Drug and remedy therapies

Dietary and postural therapies are aimed principally at correcting environmentally induced imbalances, and as such should be considered in any treatment programme where it is likely that such imbalances play a part. However, if there is an internal factor in the cause of the disease, it is unlikely that either of these two types of therapy will, on its own, be able to correct it. To correct imbalances arising internally within the organism requires the use of a therapy which can counteract such imbalances.

Homoeopathy, the Bach remedies and herbalism are all different ways of utilizing the healing properties of plants and other natural substances. The remedies seem to have the power to help harmonize the body's metabolic processes and to correct imbalances in them.

There is some debate as to the relative merits of homoeopathy and herbalism. Many plants are common to both disciplines, but the manner in which they are prescribed differs in many instances. In general, herbal remedies are prescribed for specific complaints, somewhat similar to the use of crataegus (hawthorn) in heart failure, arnica for bruising or hypericum for nerve injuries. The drug pictures (the totality of the symptoms) which are so essential for homoeopathic prescribing are not a part of herbal lore. Herbal remedies are usually dispensed as tinctures, either singly or in various combinations which are prepared specifically for the patient on the basis of their complaints.

The Bach remedies are named after their discoverer, Dr Edward Bach.[6] He was a physician who, after qualifying in medicine in 1912, worked for a time at University College Hospital, London, where he became interested in bacteriology and the developing discipline of immunology. He was intrigued by the relationships between the presence of certain abnormal intestinal bacteria which had lost the ability to ferment glucose and the diseases suffered by the patients who harboured them. He prepared vaccines from these bacteria and found that frequently a marked improvement occurred in the health of the patient after treatment by injection of the appropriate killed vaccine. Following such treatment, there was a significant change in the numbers of these organisms in the patients' bowels and this change could last for many weeks or months, during which time the patient continued to improve. He found it unwise to repeat the injections as long as the improvement was maintained.

Bach classified these bacteria into seven different groups, from each of which he prepared a vaccine, and he was able to work out the temperaments associated with each group. In many cases he was even able at the first consultation to diagnose the probable organism which the patient was harbouring on the basis of the patient's temperament, and was able to confirm these later by bacteriological studies. In 1919 he joined the staff of the London Homoeopathic Hospital as pathologist and bacteriologist, and found that he could use the homoeopathic method of potentization to prepare his vaccines which he was then able to give by mouth instead of by injection. These became known as the Bach bowel nosodes. Added to later by John Paterson, they are an important addition to the homoeopathic materia medica.

Bach also found that certain homoeopathic remedies could change the bacterial flora of patients although no conventional drugs or dietary regimes had produced any significant change. Working further on this aspect, he was able to relate certain homoeopathic remedies to certain of his bowel nosodes. He was, however, unhappy with remedies prepared from bacteria and felt that there must be plant alternatives to these which would be purer and more generally acceptable. He accordingly devoted his subsequent research efforts to discovering these plant remedies, which were to be related particularly to temperament, mood and states of mind. Bach was well aware of the effects that the mind could exert on the body, realizing that an inharmonious, negative state of mind could impair the body's vitality and reduce its ability to withstand environmental stress and insults. He particularly sought remedies which correct these negative mind states, thus freeing the patient from their harmful effects and so giving the body a better chance to heal itself.

He divided the negative states of mind into seven groups which corresponded to his seven groups of intestinal bacteria. These were: fear, indecision or uncertainty, indifference, loneliness, over-sensitivity to influences and ideas, despair or despondency and over-concern for the welfare of others. Each of these was then further subdivided so that he had a total of thirty-eight – each group corresponding to one of the thirty-eight remedies which he subsequently discovered.

These remedies are prepared from the flowers of wild plants, bushes and trees. Many of them are made by floating the freshly gathered blossoms on pure water and then allowing them to sit in the sunshine for a few hours. Some of the tree remedies, however, are prepared from flowering sprigs which include the twigs as well as the flowers and these are placed in fresh water, brought to the boil, simmered for an hour, cooled and strained. The liquids obtained by both these methods of preparation are then diluted with an equal volume of brandy, which acts as a preservative. The remedies prepared in these two ways seem to act like the high homoeopathic potencies and like these have, as their particular sphere of influence, the moods and mental states of the patient.

There are two sides to any remedy, whether it be a homoeopathic one or a Bach flower one – the positive and the negative aspects. It is the negative aspect which is used in prescribing, as this is the side which becomes apparent when the patient is ill. We should, however, never forget the positive side, which is much less well appreciated and seldom appears in the materia medica, but which is the potential for that personality type.

The Bach flower remedies and the homoeopathic remedies complement each other and can be used together in the same treatment plan. Dr Bach himself believed that his flower remedies helped to bring the physical, emotional and mental planes of the individual more into harmony with the spiritual plane and said that there could be 'no true healing unless there is a change in outlook, peace of mind and inner happiness'.

4. Electro-magnetic and related therapies

Under this heading we will consider acupuncture, electro-acupuncture, neural therapy and magnetic field therapy. In one way or another, all these therapies seem to have an effect on the electrical balances of the body.

As has already been described (Chapter 4), matter is composed of particles which may or may not be charged. All chemical and biochemical reactions depend on electrical charges and biologically active molecules carry charges which may be positive at one end of the molecule and negative at the other end. Complex, long-chain biological molecules may carry many charges, and at the cell level membranes carry charges. Such electrical charges are involved in the transport of materials across cell membranes, and in the conduction of nerve impulses. At tissue and organ level, the changing electrical patterns of the heart, muscles and brain can be recorded as electro-cardiograms (ECGs), electromyograms (EMGs) and electroencephalograms (EEGs) respectively.

The ancient Chinese believed that the electrical energy of the body flowed in specific channels known as the acupuncture meridians, and charts illustrating these have been known for several thousands of years. In the west, however, the acupuncture meridians and their accompanying acupuncture points were viewed with great scepticism and were considered to be merely figments of the imagination. After all, they did not coincide with the nerve distribution, and nerves were known to function using electrical energy.

However the use of sophisticated volt meters and resistance meters, which measure the flow of electricity in the body and degrees of block to that flow, has established the existence of both acupuncture points and acupuncture meridians. In recent years some new points and meridians have been discovered, but it is remarkable how accurate the ancient Chinese acupuncturists were.

Blocks to the flow of electrical energy in the meridians can cause problems distal to, that is, beyond, the block in organs related to that meridian. Imbalances in the electrical system can either be due to too much energy or too little energy, and acupuncture aims to correct such imbalances by removing blocks and by reducing or increasing the amount of energy. In acupuncture, needles are inserted into specific acupuncture points in order to discharge an excessive build-up of energy or to increase the amount of energy, depending on the points used. The net effect is thus to balance and harmonize the energy flow. Electro-acupuncture is a recent development in which the balancing of the energy flow is achieved by passing a weak electric current at a specific frequency – often 2.5, 10 or 80 pulses per second (Hertz or Hz) through the indicated acupuncture points. Scars across acupuncture meridians are a common source of trouble, and this can be remedied by placing electrodes on either side of the scar and treating with electro-acupuncture.

A therapy which appears to have similarities with electro-acupuncture is neural therapy, discovered in Germany in the early years of this century and also involved with electrical charges on cell membranes. In health a cell membrane has a resting potential of around +90 mV (millivolts).[7] If the cell loses its charge, it is said to be depolarized, and a cycle of depolarization and repolarization accompanies many cellular functions. If a cell becomes unable to restore its resting charge, it becomes permanently or chronically depolarized and its function is impaired.

Neural therapy aims at restoring the resting potential of depolarized cells by the injection of small amounts of local anaesthetic (procaine or xylocaine) which carries a charge of around +290 mV, and this sets off a chain of events which aids the restoration of cellular function. A number of neuromuscular conditions and conditions involving pain for no obvious reason respond well to neural therapy. A recent application in our own hands has been in the treatment of multiple sclerosis where it has been found to be of value in restoring at least some nerve function in about 60–70 per cent of patients treated. In neural therapy, the importance of scars as blocks to the flow of energy is well recognized and injection of a scar with local anaesthetic is an alternative to electro-acupuncture. Both approaches appear to achieve similar results.

Magnetic field therapy again originated in Europe and is particularly in vogue in Germany and Austria. It would appear to be similar in principle to electro-acupuncture. When electrical currents flow they produce magnetic fields and so it is possible that these two therapies amount to the same thing. The Earth's own magnetic field has a pulse frequency of 10 Hz (10 pulses/second) and it has been found that if patients are placed in magnetic fields of around 10 Hz, or are given electro-acupuncture at 10 Hz, healing can be speeded up.

Throughout the twentieth century, we have continued to increase the number of wave bands and frequencies in our environment. Radio waves, radar, television, fluorescent lights, high voltage power cables and even the electrical ring circuits in all our homes add unseen, and often unsuspected, frequencies to our environment. We have, in fact, as well as polluting our environment chemically also polluted it with radio waves of varying frequencies. The combined effects of these waves on our health and well-being are as yet unknown. It is known, however, that the immediate vicinity of a radar mast is a dangerous zone, as are the areas beneath high tension electric cables. The dangers of long exposure to fluorescent lighting and video screens are only now beginning to be appreciated, and the 50 Hz frequency of domestic electric-ring circuits may not be good news either. We know that X-rays can be extremely hazardous, and it is possible that the frequencies associated with laser printers and microwave ovens may also be suspect.

Considering that the body depends on sensitive electrical interactions to function, it would be surprising if these diverse electrical frequencies did *not* have some effect on us, whether detrimental or otherwise. It is possible, though by no means proven, that the success of magnetic fields at 10 Hz in promoting healing is simply due to a type of replacement therapy, giving the patient a good-going dose of Earth's magnetic field which has been drowned out by all the artificial, man-made frequencies surrounding us. The calming and relaxing effect of electro-acupuncture using 10 Hz through particular acupuncture points may be due to a similar reason.

Other electrical frequencies are known to have specific effects on the body. For instance, frequencies at 2–2.5 Hz stimulate the production of the body's own pain-controlling substances (the endorphins) and frequencies at around 80 Hz stimulate the production of 5 hydroxy tryptamine (serotonin), a compound involved in brain and nerve function.

5. Ego-strengthening therapies

These include relaxation therapy, hypnotherapy, auto-suggestion, autogenic training,[8] transactional analysis and meditation.

Relaxation is the basis of a number of these therapies, a

calming and a relaxing, firstly of the body and then of the emotional and mental aspects. In technique and effect, relaxation therapy, hypnosis and autohypnosis,[9] autogenic training and meditation appear to be very similar. In essence, when the body is relaxed and the mind is stilled, the brain waves (EEG) tend to run at a frequency of 7–14 Hz with a mean of 10 Hz – the same frequency as that of the Earth's magnetic field! In this state the brain is receptive to positive healing suggestions made to the patient, whether by the therapist or by the patient himself. This is termed ego-strengthening in hypnosis and several sessions of such a therapy can be very useful in helping the patient to overcome emotional, mental or even, possibly, spiritual problems. Since all levels of the individual are interrelated and interdependent, treatment on these levels can also have an effect on the physical problems, and if the root cause of the problem is on the emotional or mental plane, then treatment at this level can offer speedy relief.

Hypnosis, however, can go much further than just improving the patient's self-image. Situations can arise, whether physical, emotional, mental or spiritual, which are just too much for the individual to cope with. They are therefore eliminated from the conscious mind, in other words, forgotten, by suppressing them into the unconscious from whence, however, they continue to exert an effect. In such a case the patient is quite unaware of the root cause of the problem, because it has been successfully suppressed, and is therefore unable to help the therapist consciously with the relevant case history. In this situation, age-regression under hypnosis can be of immense value, allowing patients to free-float back under their own control to any past relevant events with which they feel they can cope, but not forcing the issue in any way. It is the belief of at least some hypnotherapists that the inability of some patients to be hypnotized is due to their subconscious fear that they will be unable to cope with what may come up and that they might go to pieces. Such an attitude on the part of the patient must be respected by the therapist.

The relationship between body posture and suppressed past trauma or emotions was touched on in the section dealing with cervical reintegration. Many people control their feelings through muscle tension and may re-experience these feelings spontaneously when the muscle spasm is broken up. Conversely, in people whose muscle spasm will not respond satisfactorily to cervical reintegration or other treatments aimed at removing muscle tension, an underlying emotional problem should be suspected.

A dramatic example of the problems with which one may be faced if the totality of the individual, with his inter-linking planes of being, is not kept in mind concerned a delegate at a hypnosis conference.[10] This man's shoulders were so stiff and tense that they practically touched his ears. At the morning coffee-break, one of his colleagues approached him and said that he practised acupuncture, and that he would relieve his shoulder tension for him if he wished. The other readily agreed; a few needles were inserted and a dramatic change in posture was quickly and effortlessly effected. All those around were greatly impressed by the power of acupuncture.

At lunch-time it was noticed that the 'patient' had disappeared, and he did not return for the start of the afternoon session. A certain amount of anxiety was felt but was relieved when he reappeared at the tea-break with his shoulders once more drawn up to his ears. He revealed to one of his colleagues that he had spent the afternoon down by a near-by river struggling with the impulse to jump in. Only by restoring his muscle spasm had he been able to conquer the impulse to commit suicide. He asked his colleague if he would consider giving him some age-regression therapy in an attempt to deal with the problem, whatever it was, that had been brought to light.

It transpired that what this man really wanted to do was to strangle his mother, a desire which was both socially and morally unacceptable and had therefore to be repressed. When the repression mechanism was removed with the acupuncture, the desire to kill had surfaced, but emerged turned against himself. When this was faced and dealt with under regression therapy, the whole situation, including the shoulder spasm, was resolved. While this case again emphasizes the links between various aspects of our being, it is also a cautionary tale underlining the possible dangers of a superficial approach to a deep-seated psychological problem.

Another interesting example of the powerful effect which hypnosis can have on the various planes of the individual is provided by the case of a middle-aged lady from Stornoway who was admitted to the local cottage hospital with terminal breast cancer. The cancer had spread from the breast to various other areas including the bones and she was as a result suffering considerable pain which was not controlled by pain-killers. She was also very much afraid. Her fear and pain combined to make her an extremely difficult patient. She was always demanding something to the extent that she completely upset the ward routine and had the nursing staff, much as they tried to sympathize with her, at the end of their tethers. It happened that one of the doctors practised hypnosis, and the sister of the ward concerned approached him and asked him if he could do anything to calm this patient who was disrupting the ward routine and upsetting the nurses. He agreed to do what he could. He had one session with the patient. He relaxed her and told her that he quite appreciated her anxiety and fear, and the fact that she was experiencing so much pain. However he assured her that she could control the pain and all she had to do to achieve this was to look at a certain corner of the ward ceiling and the pain would go. This treatment was remarkably successful. The patient was indeed able to control her pain to the extent that it completely disappeared, and her fear and anxiety disappeared as well. She became a delightful patient, no longer demanding continual attention or disturbing the ward. But not only that! Her cancer, which had not even been mentioned during the hypnosis session, rapidly regressed and after a few weeks even all radiological evidence of it had disappeared. She was discharged home, apparently fit and well, and had five years of active, happy life before she died without much pain or distress from cancer.

Hypnosis in this case relieved the patient's negative mind set and is in line with Dr Bach's thesis that such mental states, for which he developed his flower remedies, could impair the body's ability to heal itself. The relief of these negative states can have a remarkable effect on health and well-being.

Transactional analysis is a more active therapy which helps the patient to understand the basis of social interactions, and to gain insight into how to deal successfully with difficult social relationships, whether within the family or at work.

Treatment at these emotional and mental levels can of course also be obtained using homocopathy and/or Bach remedies. Different patients vary in their response to different therapies – possibly a subtle effect of the inherited background – and no therapy has yet been devised which will suit everyone.

Spiritual healing

In essence, spiritual healing is treatment aimed at correcting imbalances on the spiritual plane of being. It is, therefore, acting at the deepest level of the individual, correcting energy imbalances at the very core of our beings.

Since, as has already been shown, all planes or levels of the individual are interrelated, and imbalances or blocks at one level can affect all the others, treatment at the spiritual level can have a beneficial effect also on the mental, emotional and physical levels.

It is often not appreciated how much of the stresses and assaults that impinge upon us are suppressed into the unconscious – an area which probably lies more on the spiritual plane than the mental one. Much physical pain can be suppressed if it is too overwhelming to be borne at the time, and many emotional and mental traumas and conflicts are suppressed if they threaten the integrity or wholeness of the ego or the victim's self-image. This suppressed material, however, continues to fester away, ultimately producing imbalances and blocks on the other planes of being. Spiritual healing aims to correct these deep-seated imbalances by strengthening the flow of the life-force and removing any negative forces or imbalances. While a number of such problems can be treated successfully with deep-acting remedies or hypnotherapy, there are occasions when these cannot reach deeply enough into the patient's core. Of all the therapies available to us at the present time, spiritual healing in whatever form it is administered is probably the most deep-acting, the most misunderstood and the least often practised.

The conclusion one draws from this overview of the various therapies available is that the treatment chosen will depend on what the precipitating and underlying causes of the condition under treatment seem to be. All would appear to have their validity and their uses, and as all are concerned with either removing environmental factors or strengthening the patient's inner state, they are not in conflict and can be combined satisfactorily, often with speedier and more long-lasting results than could be obtained using only one therapy.

The enhanced results which can be obtained using a combined therapeutic regime are well illustrated by a study which we had the opportunity of carrying out about three years ago at a residential health establishment in Crieff.[11] The patients studied suffered from either osteoarthritis or rheumatoid arthritis. Treatment consisted of diet therapy, cervical reintegration and a freeze-dried preparation of the New Zealand green-lipped mussel, *Perna canaliculus*.

● The dietary regime began with a three-day wash-out period on freshly prepared fruit and vegetable juices, aimed at mobilizing toxic accumulations and eliminating them from the body. Continuing the wash-out phase, this was followed by seven days on salads, fresh vegetables and fruit – also high in fibre, vitamins, minerals and trace elements. Thereafter for the rest of their stay, which was usually two or three weeks, the patients had a fuller, wheat- and additive-free diet.

● Cervical reintegration relieved muscle tension, principally in the neck and back regions, but also locally around specific joints as indicated.

● The green-lipped mussel preparation is a remedy which, although given in material doses, is akin to homoeopathy in its mode of action. In a previous double-blind trial, it had been found to be of value in about 70 per cent of patients with rheumatoid arthritis and about 40 per cent of those with osteoarthritis.[12]

Using this combined treatment regime, the patients experienced considerable improvement in their condition in over 80 per cent of the cases, and most of this was achieved within two weeks. In some individuals the results were nothing short of spectacular. It was obvious that by using a combination of synergistic approaches to treatment, faster and better results could be obtained than with any one therapy alone.

In present-day western society, most patients will need some dietary therapy and postural correction. Thereafter the choice of acupuncture, homoeopathic or Bach remedies, neural therapy, hypnotherapy, ego-strengthening or whatever will very much depend on what the background of the illness appears to be and on the patient's response to the chosen therapy. Some patients respond quickly and satisfactorily to treatment. Others, particularly those with long-standing and deep-seated chronic diseases, may be tried with various approaches before a satisfactory response can be obtained, and some unfortunate individuals do not seem to respond well to any technique so far known. By and large, however, the more techniques available to the practitioner, the greater number of patients he or she will be able to help.

CHAPTER NINE

DOES HOMOEOPATHY

WORK?

THE RESULTS

OF RESEARCH

This chapter, like Chapter 7 (which deals with some current ideas of how homoeopathic remedies may work), is necessarily of a more scientific nature than most of the book. While every effort has been made to express the ideas in everyday language, it has been impossible to dispense with some scientific terms. Consequently the chapter is for the benefit of those with a critical interest in homoeopathy and may conveniently be glossed over by those with a less scientific turn of mind.

Despite the fact that homoeopathy has now been around for close on two hundred years, very little research has been carried out either to attempt to understand how it works, or to prove that it does work. It is tempting to suppose, however, that if homoeopathy were not efficacious it would scarcely have survived for so long, since it would be expected that doctors would cease to practise it or patients to demand it. It is true, certainly, that a number of workers who have investigated it with a view to debunking it were so impressed by the results which could be obtained with it that they became its champions instead of its detractors. Much of the so-called 'clinical evidence' for homoeopathy exists in the form of anecdotal cases which, the critics rightly point out, could easily have occurred by chance. Without some assessment of what proportion of cases are likely to respond to homoeopathic treatment, an estimate of its efficacy when compared with other therapies is impossible.

In potencies higher than the 12C, or 24X, the chances of even one molecule of the original starting material still being present are very remote. This fact, probably more than any other, has caused homoeopathy to be viewed with considerable scepticism by the orthodox 'scientific' medical profession. If there is nothing in the potency, how can you expect an effect? Any effect produced must surely be wishful thinking either on the part of the practitioner or the patient, or both.

However, in the past, many observations have been recognized to be valid before any rational or logical explanation could be advanced to account for them. Just because a thing appears to us at present to be illogical does not, of necessity, disprove its validity. With current advances in the field of physics, an explanation of the effects of homoeopathic potencies may not be too far off.

Work in the field of homoeopathic research may be divided into three broad categories:

- Investigations into the possible nature of homoeopathic potencies

- Experimental laboratory studies

- Clinical trials.

1. Investigations into the possible nature of homoeopathic potencies

Work in this field was for many years hampered by a lack of techniques sufficiently sensitive to detect changes in the solutions under study and by a rigid and over-simplified view of the nature of solutions. In considering solutions, we tend to be dominated by the idea that only the solute (the material which is dissolved) is important, and that the solvent (the substance in which the material is dissolved) is inert, apart from its ability to dissolve the solute. The idea that the solvent itself may play an important role, even when there is no demonstrable chemical reaction, has been largely neglected.

Water is the most important solvent known. It makes up 70–80 per cent of the bodies of all living things – and life as we know it would be impossible without it. All the biochemical reactions which take place in living cells take place in solution in water, or on cell organelles (small cell components) surrounded by water. Water and carbon dioxide are the two starting materials from which green plants manufacture the sugars which are themselves further elaborated by plant and animal cells into the incredible array of carbohydrates and carbohydrate-containing molecules which exist in the natural world.

In the past half century or so it has been discovered that water is a very strange substance indeed, exhibiting many anomalous and unexpected characteristics, some of which have already been mentioned in Chapter 7. We tend to accept water's anomalies unquestioningly because they are common, everyday experience. We all know that ice floats on top of the pond, though crystals forming in any other liquid would sink to the bottom. If ice did not float, pond life would not survive the winter, which means that life itself would not have survived in our climate.

It is now believed that the peculiar properties of water are due to what is known as hydrogen bonding. This means that water is not composed of individual molecules floating freely around but that the molecules are linked together. The two hydrogen atoms and the one oxygen atom which make up the water molecule form strong covalent bonds

(Figure 7, p.102). The hydrogen atoms, however, can form other weaker links with other atoms such as oxygen or nitrogen, thus linking several water molecules together. Any number of water molecules can group together in this way, giving water polymers (groups of linked molecules) of varying sizes. Polymers are formed by joining together large numbers of similar molecules, and a number have become everyday household names. Nylon, polythene, alkathene and acrilan are all polymers formed from organic molecules. The world of plastics is really a world of polymers.

Various ways of studying water strongly suggest that it is in a similar category – that is, it is a fluid containing clusters of water polymers of varying sizes[1,2] which are continually changing and reforming. The nearer the temperature is to the freezing point, the more continuous is the network of associated water molecules.[3] This has already been touched on in Chapter 7.

It has also been suggested[4] that the clustering or grouping of the water molecules will have an effect on any biological material which is dissolved in it, or which contains it. Thus the complex shapes taken up by protein molecules in the body may be due, at least in part, to the structural effects of the water. Interesting parallels have also been drawn between the vortex patterns produced by flowing water – easily seen when a thin stream of coloured water is allowed to flow into a large volume of still, clear water, or when steam rises from a hot bath – and in the whorled patterns of the horns of many animal species.[5] It is quite possible that the power of water to influence the structure of biological forms is much greater than is commonly realized.

Another intriguing aspect of water is its ability to form different crystal patterns, such as the different crystal forms of ice and snow that are produced under different weather conditions and the different ices that can be obtained under high pressures. As far back as 1949 P. W. Bridgman[6] showed that water would crystallize in a different pattern if frozen at different barometric pressures, a specific pattern being obtained for each barometric pressure.

It is against this background of a highly anomalous solvent possessing some kind of possible patterning effect that we must consider the homoeopathic potencies. These are traditionally diluted with a water/alcohol mixture – 17 per cent water, 83 per cent alcohol. Insoluble materials are firstly ground with lactose (a supposedly inert sugar with hard, abrasive crystals) to the third centesimal dilution, after which they become soluble in the water/alcohol mixture producing a colloidal solution. It is interesting that Hahnemann discovered this method of dissolving insoluble materials such as gold, silver, platinum and so on long before colloid chemistry was ever dreamt of.

Barnard[7,8] suggested that when a substance is dissolved in water or in a water/alcohol mixture, the water molecules surround each solvent molecule in a three-dimensional manner which is shape-specific for each solute – a suggestion which has been more recently substantiated.[9] He went on to say that if energy was then introduced into such a system, these shape-specific groups of water polymers could be stabilized and could join together to form long chains of water polymers which would retain the original solute imprint and shape specificity.

In the preparation of homoeopathic potencies, energy is introduced by the process of succussion in which the solution is subjected to a succession of sudden, sharp shocks. Under these conditions, water always contains some dissolved air. It has been shown[10] that if small bubbles of gas in a liquid were compressed suddenly, they would undergo very great temperature changes of the order of several thousand degrees centigrade. Some of the water molecules would be split at such a temperature and would be available for chemical or physical activity as soon as the bubble burst. It is considered that this phenomenon explains the excessive corrosion around ships' propellers, and the finding of nitric acid in trace amounts in pure water passing through small apertures at high pressure. It may also explain the occurrence of nitrogen fixation around sea shores where there is constant turbulence produced by the waves continually breaking on the shore.

Barnard considered that the energy introduced into the homoeopathic potency during the succussion process stabilized the arrangement of the water polymers and that it was these shape-specific polymers which were built up and passed on from one potency to the next. He also postulated that when they reached a certain length they fractured, producing several shorter lengths of shape-specific polymer which then continued to grow again as the potentization process was continued. On this theory some potencies would contain more shape-specific molecules than others and some would contain longer chain polymers than others, so some potencies might be expected to be more efficacious than others in treatment. The shape-specific polymers continued to be passed on from potency to potency even after none of the original solute was left in the solution. Barnard's observation that succussed solutions showed a greater viscosity than the equivalent simple dilutions prepared without succussion provides some evidence that homoeopathic potencies do indeed contain long-chain molecules.

Further evidence for macro-molecules comes from the work of Heintz[11] who obtained infra-red absorption patterns of succussed solutions which indicated that polymers were produced in the solvent. The effect was not uniform over all the potencies but showed peaks and troughs of activity, with some potencies showing more absorption than others (Figure 11). This peaking effect was destroyed by boiling the solutions, a process which might be expected

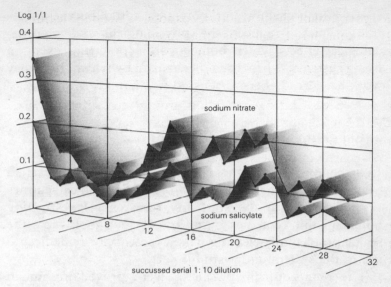

Figure 11. Infra-red absorption spectra of succussed solutions of sodium nitrate and sodium salicylate

to destroy long-chain water polymers. No peaking was observed in simple dilutions prepared without succussion.

Both the infra-red absorption studies of Heintz and the viscosity studies of Barnard have yet to be repeated by other workers, but they are both suggestive of the presence of polymers in the potencies. Similar conclusions can be drawn from nuclear magnetic-spin resonance studies[12] – work which also requires verification.

The increasingly sensitive techniques now available offer an unparalleled opportunity for fuller research into the nature of homoeopathic potencies. It is to be hoped that if a well-proven scientific basis for potency action is established, much of the scepticism towards homoeopathy will disappear. The results obtained so far suggest that shape-

specific long-chain water polymers could be the something which produces the physiological and pharmacological effects which homoeopathic potencies exert on
living systems. A proposed mechanism by which these may
work has already been discussed in Chapter 7.

2. Experimental laboratory studies

In orthodox medicine these studies are traditionally carried
out using plants, animals, micro-organisms and cell culture
systems. Right at the start any researcher investigating
homoeopathic remedies by means of such tools faces the
major problem of selecting which remedy, or remedies, to
use in the system under study.

The homoeopathic potencies were proved in human
volunteers, and information was collected on the physical,
emotional, mental and psychological changes experienced
by the provers. The totality of the symptoms, including the
very important emotional and mental characteristics, are
the pointers for remedy selection. In animals physical and
emotional, if not mental, changes do occur but these have
to be elicited by careful observation of the animal, as it is
not easy for it to indicate directly how it feels, or how its
perceptions and emotions have changed. However homoeopathy is very successful in veterinary practice and it is
theoretically possible that suitable animal tests could be
devised for the study of at least some homoeopathic
remedies.

When it comes to plants, micro-organisms and tissue
culture systems, the remedy picture as worked out for
human patients is wholly inappropriate, and experiments
have to be conducted on the basis of trial and error to see if
particular remedies have an effect on particular plants or
micro-organisms. The failure of such experiments to

demonstrate any effect of homoeopathic remedies is therefore just as likely to be due to inappropriate remedy
selection for the model under study as to the possibility
that the remedy really is inactive, or that homoeopathy is
just a load of fantasy, wishful thinking and mumbo jumbo.

Despite these difficulties, however, a number of workers
have successfully demonstrated effects of homoeopathic
remedies under experimental conditions. One of the earliest
workers in this field was L. Kolisko[13] in Switzerland, who
published the results of her observations of various
potencies on plant growth in 1923. Her experiments showed
peaks and troughs of activity with different potencies, similar to the infra-red absorption spectra later demonstrated
by Heintz and postulated by Barnard's theory. These results were confirmed by Dr W. E. Boyd's meticulous work
in Glasgow,[14] using potencies of mercuric chloride and the
enzyme diastase, which converts starch to sugar. Mercuric
chloride was selected because it is a growth inhibitor, and
Boyd found that homoeopathically prepared potencies of
mercuric chloride enhanced the speed at which the diastase
converted the starch when compared with controls which
did not contain the mercuric chloride potency. It was interesting that the growth inhibitor, in potency, stimulated
the activity of the enzyme. The experiments were repeated
many times with similar results which were highly significant statistically.

Both Kolisko's and Boyd's experiments were painstaking
and proved to be impossible for other workers to replicate
because of the complicated experimental apparatus
involved. Some investigators[15,16,17] obtained conflicting
results using copper chloride and iron sulphide potencies
on cress seedlings, and some[18,19] claimed effects with
mercuric chloride on lymphoblasts (a type of white blood
cell) in tissue culture, an effect not substantiated by
others.[20] Accelerated growth of algae partially poisoned

with copper sulphate has been claimed when these were treated with a 30th potency of copper sulphate,[21,22] but Moss[23] was not able to repeat this work. He, however,[24] did find that some potentized remedies showed effects on the macrophages (white cells) of some batches of guinea-pigs but not in others, and in the macrophages of one human subject but not in others. These results are in line with the knowledge that not everyone will respond to the same remedy, as some individuals are more sensitive to a remedy than others for whom it is not indicated. These conflicting experimental results may in fact be indicating that different batches or strains of the same species of plant, too, may exhibit different reaction patterns to the same homoeopathic remedy, and serve to underline the difficulty of using animal or plant models in a situation where, even with a cooperative patient giving a good history, remedy selection can be extremely difficult.

Perhaps some of the most encouraging experimental results started with the work carried out in Switzerland by W. Pelikan and G. Unger, and published in English in 1965.[25] These workers reported the effects of various potencies of silver nitrate (*Argentum nitricum*) on the growth of wheat seedlings which gave reproducible results over an experimental period of about a year. Using potencies from 8X to 19X they obtained graphs of growth against potency with peaks and troughs reminiscent of those obtained by Kolisko and predicted by Barnard's theory. This work was confirmed by R. L. Jones and M. D. Jenkins in London,[26] using a number of different remedies including silver nitrate, arnica, potassium carbonate (*Kali carbonicum*), actea racemosa, bryonia and nux vomica on the growth of wheat seedlings. There were significant differences between the controls and some of the potencies, and the results were reproducible. Over the potency range of 6C to 24C of arnica, plots of growth against potency produced similar graphs with peaks and troughs of growth response.

These same authors went on to compare the effects of homoeopathic potencies on the wheat seedlings with those on cultures of yeast, and obtained very similar results.[27] They concluded that yeast provided just as reliable an experimental model as wheat, with the advantage of quicker growth and therefore faster results. Using the yeast model, they have demonstrated different effects with different degrees of succussion and have also shown that the rest period between finishing the succussion of one potency and sampling it for dilution to prepare the next potency is important.[28] The results to date would seem to indicate that a rest period of at least three minutes is required between one dilution and the next. Perhaps this length of time is required for the long-chain polymers to stabilize after the succussion process ends.

Whereas these workers have successfully repeated their own experiments, others in Yorkshire[29] have been unable to do so. In these latter experiments, however, a different strain of yeast was used from that employed by Jones and Jenkins, and it may well be that this is another example of one strain of an organism being more sensitive to particular homoeopathic remedies than others. Additionally, with the exception of silver nitrate, the remedies tested in these latter experiments were different from those tested by Jones and Jenkins, and it may be that a less appropriate selection was made.

Less work has been done with animal models, but recent work from India[30] has shown that some homoeopathic remedies in various potencies displayed anti-viral activity in developing chick embryos, whereas other remedies had no anti-viral effect in mice.

Experiments with animals are not a feature of homoeopathic research and many people feel that it is ethical to carry out such studies only if the animals are to benefit, as in veterinary medicine. However, some limited studies using animals have been carried out in France. Work undertaken in 1955[31] showed that potentized arsenic could increase the excretion of arsenic by arsenic-poisoned guinea-pigs. More recently[32] work from the Boiron Laboratories in Lyon has suggested that a 7C potency of *Arsenicum album* caused a significant excretion of arsenic by arsenic-poisoned rats as compared with a 7C potency of water used as a control, thus confirming the earlier observations with the guinea-pigs.

This idea of using a homoeopathic potency of a poison to counteract the effects of that poison – in other words, isopathy – has been extended to study the effects of potencies of mercury in mercury poisoning. Using mercury-poisoned human skin fibroblasts (fibrous tissue cells) in culture, the Boiron workers obtained protective effects with some potencies of *Mercurius corrosivus* as compared with water potentized to the same level.[33]

Other work carried out in the Boiron Laboratories[34] provides suggestive evidence that gelsemium in both tincture and potency can affect the speed with which chemicals which transmit nerve impulses are inactivated in the brain. This is interesting work which suggests other possible lines of research since gelsemium (jasmine) is an extremely poisonous plant which affects the central nervous system, giving rise to muscular quiverings and cramps and problems with coordination, followed later by paralysis.

Gelsemium, in its provings, has aching of the muscles and stiffness in the neck region, weakness and trembling of the limbs, shivers and chills, occipital headache, double vision, dullness and apathy. Stage fright, loss of memory and diarrhoea are also part of the picture. Gelsemium would thus seem to be an appropriate choice of remedy to use in neurological experiments.

In the field of allergic reactions, homoeopathic potencies of histamine (histaminum 7C) and honey bee (*Apis mellifica*) were studied for their effect on the degranulation of basophils. Basophils are one type of white blood cell and their granules contain histamine which is one of the substances involved in the production of allergic reactions. Degranulation of the basophils occurs in immediate hypersensitivity reactions (one type of allergic reaction), releasing the histamine which is responsible for a number of the features of such reactions.

The French workers[35] found that the potencies of histaminum and *Apis mellifica* could prevent the degranulation of allergen-sensitized basophils when they were incubated with the appropriate allergen. This action may well underlie the use of these remedies to treat generalized allergic reactions and bee stings respectively.

Though not so far repeated by other workers elsewhere, this French work would seem to demonstrate test-tube (*in vitro*) effects of homoeopathic potencies, albeit low ones, in a wide variety of laboratory situations. The models used are well chosen for the remedies studied and could stimulate the development of further experiments along similar lines.

Another potentially useful system for laboratory study could well be the various steps in prostaglandin synthesis. In view of the wide effects that defects in this metabolic system can have on the body, they may well be suited to study of the polychrests – that is, the remedies with a wide sphere of action such as *Natrum muriaticum*, silica, sepia, lycopodium, sulphur, phosphorus or lachesis to name but a few.

3. Clinical trials

Although homoeopathy has been practised for nearly two hundred years in many countries of the world, very little work has been performed in the way of well-conducted clinical trials to prove and assess its efficacy. One reason for this is undoubtedly the fact that many of those who are attracted to homoeopathy are well content just to treat patients as they present, and do not have the expertise or the scientific bent of mind required to design and carry out clinical trials.

Another reason is the difficulty experienced in designing a well-controlled homoeopathic trial. In conventional trials set up to to assess the efficacy of a new drug, the drug is given to a group of patients suffering from a particular illness, and the effects are compared with those obtained in a matched group of patients given a dummy (or placebo) drug. The design is relatively simple because in orthodox practice the treatment is determined by the category of illness. The same drug can therefore be used for all cases of the condition, although even in conventional medicine not all patients will respond to it.

In the homoeopathic approach, on the other hand, the treatment is determined not by the condition from which the patient is suffering but from his or her reaction to that condition, the totality of the symptom picture. A homoeopathic physician is therefore likely to use a number of different remedies in the treatment of any particular condition. Indeed, the same patient may require more than one remedy at different stages of the treatment programme. Conversely, the same remedy may be used to treat several different clinical conditions if the patients suffering from them respond in a similar way to their illnesses. It is therefore impracticable to carry out a trial of a single homoeopathic remedy versus a single orthodox drug or placebo, although this approach has been tried. On the other hand, to conduct a trial of homoeopathy as a whole versus placebo or an orthodox drug brings its own problems and criticisms.

A simpler situation to study is that of allergy. In allergy the condition can be treated with a potency of the substance to which the patient is allergic, such as house dust in cases of house-dust-mite allergy, grass pollens in hay fever, chloroform in chloroform allergy (as in the case of the technician described in Chapter 1) and so on. In these situations the same remedy is appropriate for all cases of the condition.

A few years ago,[36] an assessment was made of the efficacy of treating house-dust-mite, allergic patients with a combination of mite exclusion and the 200C potency of house dust. This was not a controlled trial but a retrospective assessment of the patients seen over the previous seven years. Nor was it an assessment of homoeopathy alone, but of homoeopathy in combination with avoidance of exposure to the sensitizing organism.

The results of this combined treatment, however, were very encouraging, with 85 per cent of children and 79 per cent of adults benefiting from this approach. Early on in the running of the clinic it had been found that treatment with house dust 200 alone was less effective and less long-lasting if the avoidance programme was not also undertaken, but it was not possible, from the nature of the study, to assess what proportion of the benefit was attributable to each measure.

A more recent study[37] in the allergy field was a double-blind placebo-controlled pilot trial of the efficacy of mixed pollen 30C in hay fever. The results of this trial were encouraging, the benefits of the potency reaching statistical significance. A later follow-up trial showed similar results.[38]

Despite the increased difficulties, trials have been carried out on the effects of homoeopathy in a chronic condition – rheumatoid arthritis. In a pilot trial[39] the results of treatment with homoeopathy in a group of patients were compared with the results of aspirin treatment in a slightly smaller, but otherwise similar group. After a year, the homoeopathically treated group was substantially better than the aspirin group, with two thirds of the patients better than they had been at the start of the trial, while none of the patients on aspirin had improved and most of them had dropped out, either because of unacceptable side-effects, or because the treatment was ineffective.

This trial was followed up with a double-blind, placebo-controlled trial[40,41] in which twenty-three patients given homoeopathy were compared with twenty-three matched patients given placebo; all patients being, in addition, on standard conventional non-steroidal anti-inflammatory drugs – these being matched in the two groups. Significant improvements were obtained in stiffness, pain and functional ability in the homoeopathically treated group compared with the placebo group. There were no improvements in the placebo group despite the fact that the patients were on full orthodox first-line treatment.

A more recent trial in osteoarthritis[42] showed no effect from *Rhus toxicodendron* when compared with placebo. This trial was an attempt to use the orthodox model, comparing a single remedy with placebo. The parameters used to select patients for the trial, however, could have indicated several remedies other than *Rhus toxicodendron*, and the chances of any particular patient responding to the *Rhus toxicodendron* were little better than might have been expected by chance alone. In such a trial, with the numbers of patients involved, it would have been surprising if a statistically significant effect of *Rhus toxicodendron* *had* been demonstrated.

The situation at the moment in the field of research in homoeopathy is that much encouraging and interesting work demonstrating effects of homoeopathic potencies has been carried out in a wide variety of laboratory and clinical models. The fact that work performed by one group is not necessarily found to be repeatable by another is nothing new. Much laboratory work carried out in other fields is found to be irrepeatable by other workers and many orthodox drug trials also produce conflicting results. One reason for this may well be the inability of other laboratories to reproduce exactly the conditions under which the initial observations were made. Any living system is highly complex and subject to many environmental influences, some of which are probably totally unrecognized. Factors as subtle as the weather, time of year and phases of the moon – to which varying individual responses form part of the drug pictures of a number of homoeopathic remedies – may well play a part.

Inherited factors are also important. It always has to be borne in mind in orthodox research that while strains of laboratory animals are highly inbred to ensure, as far as possible, consistency of response, complete homogeneity can never be guaranteed, and genetic similarity is even less likely to be achieved with plants. When it comes to the more subtle realms of responses and sensitivities to homoeopathic remedies, even small strain variations could so change the sensitivity of the species under study that one strain might respond well to a particular remedy while a second, apparently similar strain may not respond at all. This problem may well underlie many of the conflicting results obtained from plant experiments.

Should it become necessary, to meet EEC requirements on medicines legislation, to run tests with homoeopathic remedies using double-blind models, the great advantage of research with the remedies is their gentle action and lack of the harmful side-effects which unfortunately result from many orthodox drugs.

A further factor which can have an effect on the results of an experiment is the mental attitude of the experimenter.

Expectation has been shown to influence the outcome of even the most carefully controlled double-blind trial[43] in either a positive or a negative direction. Such mental attitudes may be wholly unconscious and are difficult, if not impossible, to eliminate.

The research carried out so far has established some useful ideas and models which could be more intensively investigated and has established guidelines for future clinical trials. Further refinements in technique and trial design may well open the way for much exciting and profitable research in homoeopathy in the near future.

CHAPTER TEN

QUESTIONS

AND ANSWERS

Because homoeopathy tends to be unfamiliar to the majority of people, they ask a lot of questions about it. Over the years it has become apparent that certain questions are asked more often than others. We have collected together a representative sample of these and present them here. Although many of them have been answered already in an expanded form elsewhere in the book, we are including them again here in a more concise form for easy reference.

1. What is homoeopathy?

Homoeopathy is a process of natural healing in which the remedies are used to assist the body to heal itself by stimulating its natural healing powers. The name is derived from two Greek words and means the treating of like with like. This means that when one is treating a patient with homoeopathy, a substance is used which produces in a healthy person symptoms and signs similar to those presented by that patient.

2. What kind of substances are used?

The remedies used in homoeopathy are in the main derived from the mineral, vegetable and animal kingdoms. More rarely, disease products from specific diseases such as measles, chicken pox, whooping cough, syphilis, gonorrhoea, cancer etc. are used to produce the corresponding nosode. The latter are sometimes necessary to clear either the after-effects of these infections or inherited traits passed on from infected forebears before other remedies can work to clear up the case. In specific instances remedies can be made from particular antigens if the remedy is not already present in the materia medica, or from particular orthodox drugs if patients have a sensitivity to these. Examples of these are chloroform, penicillin and cortisone.

3. How does homoeopathy work?

The short answer to this question is that we do not know how homoeopathic remedies work any more than we know how the majority of orthodox pharmaceuticals work. It is postulated, however, that the remedies may key into the body's basic metabolism, possibly harmonizing immune reactions or smoothing out difficulties in the basic mechanisms controlling body function. The action depends on the ability of the remedy to stimulate the body to produce a healing response – or, to put it another way, on the body's ability to mount a healing response. If the body's vitality is low, or if its reactive powers have been suppressed through long exposure to steroid drugs, homoeopathic remedies are often ineffective.

4. How is homoeopathy different from the orthodox medicine I can get from my GP?

Orthodox medicines tend to be palliative rather than curative. They help the patient by easing the symptoms or by replacing substances such as hormones or vitamins which are deficient in the body. Homoeopathy, on the other hand, stimulates the body to heal itself and its use can be truly curative. The two systems are therefore working from different standpoints.

5. I am concerned about the side-effects associated with some orthodox drugs. Does homoeopathic medicine have these?

No, homoeopathy is not associated with toxic side-effects. Although many of the homoeopathic remedies are poisons in their crude form, the process of potentization by which homoeopathic remedies are prepared separates the healing power of the remedy – the quality of the remedy – from the toxic effects, which are associated with the quantity. The remedies, therefore, do not have side-effects in the accepted sense of the word.

They can, however, produce an aggravation. This is an intensification of the patient's symptoms and signs and it can be unpleasant, or even alarming, for the patient. It tends to happen if too high a potency (that is, too strong a potency) is given, and the symptoms are brought out or exteriorized rather too quickly for the body to handle comfortably. The symptoms are moving in the opposite direction to suppression and this is necessary if a long-lasting cure is to be achieved. An aggravation is usually short-lived, and even when present the patient often feels better. It is usually followed by a substantial improvement in the patient's condition.

6. Does an aggravation happen in every case?
No. Ideally the cure should be effected without producing an aggravation. Where an aggravation is produced, the optimum potency has not been given and the symptoms have been brought out too rapidly for the body to be able to handle harmoniously. Too high a potency, with too much energy, has been given, rather like using a sledge-hammer to crack a nut when a simple nut-cracker would have been more appropriate. The end result, however, is usually beneficial as the aggravation is normally followed by a healing response.

7. How long has homoeopathic medicine been in existence?
Homoeopathy has been around for nearly two hundred years. It was formulated by Dr Samuel Hahnemann, a German physician, about the year 1806. The principle of

treatment of like by like, however, had been enunciated by Hippocrates in the fifth century BC, but it had been forgotten for centuries until rediscovered by Hahnemann.

8. What started it?

History relates that it all began when Hahnemann was translating a treatise on materia medica written by the Scottish physician Dr William Cullen, a section of which dealt with the use of cinchona bark (otherwise known as Peruvian bark) from which we obtain quinine to treat malaria. Hahnemann disagreed with Cullen's hypothesis as to the mode of action of cinchona and took some himself to see what effect it would have. To his surprise he discovered that it produced in him the symptoms and signs of the illness which it was used to treat, namely malaria, which in those days was known as intermittent fever. Hahnemann then went on from this to study the effects in healthy people of other medicinal substances, and having documented these effects used the substances to treat people suffering from those patterns of symptoms and signs. From the results of these studies, he enunciated the principle that like cures like.

9. Has it changed much since Hahnemann's time?

Since then, the homoeopathic materia medica has been expanded considerably as more and more remedies are proved. New nosodes have also been added to the armamentarium and special remedies prepared from specific antigens and toxic substances. The principles of homoeopathy, as laid down by Hahnemann, are as valid today as they were in his time. Various schools of thought, however, have evolved, with the low potency school of Hughes and the high potency school of Kent being the main contenders in this country. In Latin America other schools of thought have arisen, such as those of Masi and Orthega, but it is yet to be demonstrated that they are any more effective than the guidelines laid down by Hahnemann in the sixth edition of his *Organon of Rational Healing*.

10. Can homoeopathic medicines be used to treat all kinds of conditions?

Yes, within limits. There is no class of disease in which homoeopathy cannot be used, although if the case has reached the stage of requiring surgery, for instance, this should not be delayed. Depending on how much irreversible damage has, or has not, occurred, the results of homoeopathic treatment may range from minimal to spectacular. In injuries and accidents, the injury remedies can be of great value, and even when surgery is indicated they can be helpful in shortening the post-operative period and in speeding up the recovery process.

11. Can homoeopathy help with allergies?

Yes, very definitely. The use of the potentized allergen is, in most cases, very successful in relieving the symptoms of allergy. For a deeper cure this can be followed up with the constitutional remedy.

12. Can homoeopathy help with chronic disease?

Again the answer is yes. In many cases homoeopathic treatment is much more successful than orthodox treatment and can achieve results which would be considered impossible with orthodox treatment. Much of this success is due to the ability of homoeopathic remedies to treat precipitating factors, however far back in the patient's medical history, and inherited predispositions.

13. Can homoeopathy help with life-threatening conditions – for example, cancer?

Cancer is by no means the only life-threatening condition. Many acute life-threatening conditions, shock states etc. are eminently treatable with homoeopathy. When it comes to cancer, a multidisciplinary approach is often the most successful. Any possible environmental factors, with emphasis on diet, should always be dealt with. Homoeopathy can certainly help to improve the body's function and the anthroposophical remedy iscador – prepared from mistletoe and similar to *Viscum album* in the homoeopathic materia medica – can be helpful in certain types of cancer. However, many cancers are not amenable to treatment on these levels alone. Although homoeopathy can work deeply into the organism, and can affect the deeper emotional, mental and spiritual levels, therapies more specifically aimed at developing the spiritual aspects of human beings may well be needed in addition as the root of the cancer problem often lies at this level. Creative meditation techniques can be of great value here.

14. Does homoeopathy avoid the need for surgery?
The answer to this question very much depends on how far the illness has gone. If it has got to the length of requiring surgery, then certainly surgery should not be delayed. Ideally, of course, one hopes to get the case before it has reached this stage. Then, if the choice of remedy is correct, the need for surgery should be obviated.

15. If one has to have surgery can homoeopathy help?
Yes, certainly it can. Remedies can be given both pre-operatively and post-operatively to speed up healing and to counteract any effects of anxiety, shock and the anaesthetic. In general, patients treated with homoeopathy make a much more rapid post-operative recovery than patients who have not had this treatment.

16. Is homoeopathy safe for babies and children?
Yes, since there are no toxic effects. Additionally, since babies and young children often have a high level of vitality, excellent results are to be expected.

17. What happens if a child inadvertently swallows a lot of homoeopathic tablets?

It does not matter. Such a situation would be treated by the body as a single dose. If the remedy is not indicated it will be ignored by the body and will have no effect, and if it is indicated it can only be beneficial. It is only when a remedy is taken over an extended period that proving symptoms are likely to occur.

18. Do homoeopathic physicians prescribe antibiotics?

Yes, they do. Where an antibiotic is indicated, it is negligent for a doctor not to prescribe it. However the homoeopathic physician will also administer a remedy, as well as giving a prescription for the antibiotic, with instructions that should the remedy not have worked within an hour or two, the antibiotic should be obtained. In most instances, if the correct remedy is given, the antibiotic will not be required.

19. Can homoeopathy help older people to remain mentally and physically active for longer?

This is a difficult question to answer. Individuals who seek homoeopathic treatment tend, on the whole, to be open-minded and willing to recognize the relationships between man and nature. Such individuals, because of their active interests and state of mind, do tend to live longer than those who are not so active and aware, but whether this can be ascribed to homoeopathic treatment or whether it is a spin-off of their state of mind is a moot point.

20. Can you be treated with homoeopathy if you are already being treated with orthodox medicine?

Yes, usually there is no conflict between the two approaches. In the rheumatology trials which we carried out, all the patients were on orthodox first-line anti-inflammatory drugs at the start of the trials, though after treatment a number were able to discontinue these. Most of the patients seen at the hospital and the out-patient clinics are already on conventional medication of some kind. The only rider to this is the prolonged use of steroids and drugs which have an effect on the body's immune system as these damp down the body's ability to react and often render subsequent homoeopathic treatment difficult.

21. Should I tell my doctor that I am also having homoeopathic medicine?

Yes, you should. In the first place, if you are being seen in a hospital out-patient department, the doctor who sees you should write to your GP to inform him of what treatment has been given. Secondly, it is only right that your doctor should know, because if there is a significant change in your condition with homoeopathy, he will ascribe it to the wrong treatment if he does not know that other therapies have also been given.

22. Can I get homoeopathy on the NHS?

Yes. Homoeopathy has been a part of the NHS since its inception in 1948. Unfortunately, however, there are not enough homoeopathic doctors to meet the demand for this form of treatment and many areas of the country do not have a homoeopathic practitioner.

23. Is it expensive if I have to have it privately?

This varies quite a bit, depending on the training and experience of the practitioner. However, clinics such as the Manchester Homoeopathic Clinic are run very reasonably and other clinics are being developed at present along similar lines. But, as an initial consultation may be as long as one hour, charges have to be pitched accordingly.

24. How do I find out where to get homoeopathy?

The Faculty of Homoeopathy produces a list of all homoeopathic doctors practising in this country and abroad with indications as to whether they are private or NHS practitioners. This booklet is available at the

Faculty headquarters and also at the various homoeopathic hospitals and clinics around the country. By sending a letter enclosing a stamped addressed envelope to one of these centres, you can find out who and where your nearest practitioner is. See Appendix 3 for useful addresses.

25. Is a consultation with a homoeopathic doctor anything like a visit to an ordinary GP?

Not really. The homoeopathic doctor needs to obtain a large amount of information from the patient which requires a longer consultation time. In an NHS clinic this may be only ten to fifteen minutes, but the average practitioner seeing a patient privately likes to give about an hour to the first interview, so that a good idea of as many facets of the patient as possible can be ascertained. Many of the questions asked may surprise the newcomer to homoeopathy as they are not ones that a GP usually asks. Any clinical examination required will be similar to that carried out by the ordinary GP.

26. Are the medicines expensive and where do you get them? How often do you have to take them?

The medicines are not expensive. The cost varies but the average homoeopathic prescription to buy privately costs less, and in some cases a lot less, than the standard NHS prescription charge. The number of times you have to take the medicines varies: frequently in an acute condition and less frequently in a chronic one. For where to get the medicines see the list of useful addresses in Appendix 3.

27. Can you use homoeopathy for first aid and self-help in the home? If so, how can I learn about this?

Homoeopathy is eminently suitable for first aid and self-help treatment. Its use in accident situations and acute emergencies is much simpler than prescribing for long-term chronic conditions. Under the auspices of the British Homoeopathic Association, a home remedy kit has been developed with remedies for acute situations and instructions on how to use them. They include injury remedies and remedies for acute fevers, diarrhoea and vomiting, frights, shocks and other acute and sudden conditions. When these are issued to patients with the instructions, it is found that the amount of acute visiting required is cut down considerably. These kits really are a must for any home medicine cabinet. For details on where to obtain them see Appendix 3.

28. Are the medicines prepared in a special way?

Yes. Great care has to be taken in the preparation of homoeopathic remedies to avoid contamination and the plants used have to be grown under organic conditions, well away from any possible environmental pollution. The processes of dilution and succussion are specific to homoeopathy and are not used in the preparation of any other forms of medicine, although somewhat similar methods are used by the anthroposophical people in the preparation of the Weleda range of remedies and products.

29. Is homoeopathy scientific?

Homoeopathy is based on the observations which resulted from a number of studies and on further experimental investigations derived from these. In this respect, although usually referred to as empirical, it can be considered to be scientific. The fact that laboratory studies and clinical trials now exist to confirm its efficacy validate this claim.

30. How does homoeopathy differ from herbalism?

Many of the same plants are used in both herbalism and homoeopathy but the prescribing indications can be very different. Another difference is that herbal medicines are not subjected to the potentization process, as is done in homoeopathy, but are given in material doses, often as tinctures. Homoeopathic remedies can also be administered in the form of tinctures, but when material doses are called for, a 3X or 6X potency is more often given. Again, many herbal prescriptions will contain more than one remedy. It does not seem to matter if these are mixed together in the one preparation whereas in classical homoeopathy it is held that remedies should not be mixed. If more than one remedy is indicated, in classical homoeopathy it is believed that they should be administered separately to allow the body to process each one individually. On the continent, however, mixtures are used, though how effective this is compared with single remedy prescriptions is still to be evaluated.

31. Can homoeopathy help in pregnancy?

Yes. Many of the common problems of pregnancy such as simple morning sickness, hyperemesis, urinary infections and so on, are eminently treatable with homoeopathy which is particularly indicated in pregnancy, since there is no risk of toxic effects which might harm the foetus. In the last month of pregnancy, caulophyllum is given to prepare the muscles and ligaments of the birth canal for an easy delivery. Caulophyllum is also known as squaw root because it was used by the Red Indian squaws to achieve easy childbirth.

32. Is there a homoeopathic alternative to vaccination and immunization?

Yes. The nosodes of the specific diseases can be used as a preventative in this way – for instance, morbillinum for measles, pertussin for whooping cough, variolinum for smallpox, tuberculinum for tuberculosis and so on. Belladonna, which is not a nosode, may clear up and prevent scarlet fever, though this disease is little seen nowadays. Pulsatilla, which also is not a nosode, can be useful in both the treatment and prevention of measles. These remedies were used to protect children from these diseases in the days before the vaccination and immunization schedules were developed. Unfortunately, no trials of efficacy were carried out at that time, and this is impossible to do now as the vaccination schedules are in such widespread use. Hard data on the degree of protection afforded by the homoeopathic remedies, therefore, does not exist. Nevertheless, anecdotal clinical experience would suggest that they are effective and, again, they are not associated with harmful side-effects.

33. When taking the medicines do I have to change my diet, give up smoking and/or drinking?

This is a regular old chestnut and the advice given depends very much on who is giving it. We ourselves have found that if a patient goes on to a diet which is relatively free from pesticides, herbicides and chemical additives, then often the homoeopathic remedies work much better than if the patient continues to eat an additive and junk-food-laden diet. This probably also holds for smoking and drinking. However, these two activites tend to be associated with addictions and personality difficulties in the patient and to require them to give up these things can often be counterproductive, since compliance may well bring on a withdrawal syndrome, and failure can lead to anxiety and guilt. It is to be hoped that as the patient begins to feel better, there will be less need for either smoking or alcohol. In some instances, patients are able to discontinue these habits themselves without much difficulty later on. An example of this is the young man with the enlarged spleen whose story was told in Chapter 1.

Some homoeopathic practitioners advise that patients should not drink coffee, or even tea, while under homoeopathic treatment, as it is considered that coffee in particular tends to inactivate the remedies. This may well be true, though at present there is no hard evidence for it. If patients wish to give up coffee, it is perhaps not a bad thing. Some instant coffees are associated with problems similar to wheat-sensitivity in a number of patients and are better avoided along with wheat.

34. How can such a diluted form of medicine be so powerful?

We believe that the homoeopathic remedies are an information system and, as such, depend for their action on the *quality* of the remedy rather than on its *quantity*. Information systems in the body act at subtle levels in minute, trace amounts and the scale of the homoeopathic remedies is in keeping with much of what we now know about biological integrating and controlling mechanisms.

35. Can homoeopathy be used in conjunction with other forms of alternative medicine?

Certainly. Often if various different approaches are used, a much faster and longer-lasting result is obtained. For instance, in a group of patients with rheumatoid and osteo arthritis who were treated with an elimination diet followed by a wheat-free diet, cervical reintegration and the green-lipped mussel preparation, Seatone, significant and often dramatic improvements were obtained in a fortnight of an order similar to, or better than, those obtained by either homoeopathy or Seatone alone over a period of three to six months. Most forms of alternative medicine work harmoniously and synergistically together to produce combined effects which are often greater than the sum of the individual effects attributable to each.

At present we ourselves consider that any treatment programme, whether homoeopathic or otherwise, should start off with attention to diet. This will facilitate whatever remedy treatment is to be given. Consideration should also be given to posture and exercise. Bach remedies are often given along with homoeopathic remedies and any other therapies such as acupuncture, magnetic field therapy, neural therapy and so on can be added in as indicated.

36. What is meant by treating you as a whole person?
This means that the practitioner recognizes that the patient is not just a physical entity but also has emotional, mental and spiritual aspects – all or any of which may need treatment. It is also recognized that this complex individual does not live in isolation but is in continual interaction with his or her environment, and that this must also be taken into account in both assessing the problem and planning the treatment.

37. If homoeopathy is such an individual way of treating you – for example, one person with influenza may have quite a different medicine from another person with it – what is the value of homoeopathic remedies now seen on many chemists' shelves which could be used by people who are not aware that the choice of a remedy has to be selected according to a number of factors, not just by a simple set of symptoms?
Firstly, it is inadvisable to take remedies consisting of mixtures as no homoeopathic provings have been done on mixtures and it is not known whether the effects of these are different from the effects of their individual components. Provided that the instructions on the indications for such remedies as the tissue salts are carefully followed, and that they are not taken for long periods, they may be of benefit. If taken over an extended period, however, patients may start to prove these remedies but fail to realize that new symptoms which they are beginning to experience are linked to the remedy which they are taking. The injury remedies such as arnica have easy and specific indications. In the case of the home remedy kits full instruction for use, with the specific indications, are supplied.

38. What is meant by the Schussler tissue salts?

These are a group of twelve low potency (3X to 12X) homoeopathic remedies prepared from inorganic salts which were found, in the early days of homoeopathy, to be present in the blood and tissue fluids. Dr Schussler, who had a particular interest in physiology, considered that a number of diseases were due to a deficiency of one or more of these salts and thought that if a patient exhibited the symptoms of a remedy – for instance *Natrum muriaticum* – there was a deficiency of this salt in the patient's body. He found that by giving the salt in low potency there was often an improvement in the patient's well-being.

Inevitably, since there are only twelve tissue salt preparations, an attempt was made with varying degrees of success to enlarge their scope by mixing them in an effort to cover other symptomatologies. The problem with the mixtures is that they have never been proved in the classical homoeopathic way, as had been done with the original remedies. More recent biochemical studies demonstrate that many more inorganic elements occur in the body than those which make up the twelve tissue salts. Schussler attempted, with his salts, to simplify homoeopathy to make it easier to practise, but his concept of deficiency disease has not been validated and his ideas are not in line with classical homoeopathic principles.

Another problem is that if the remedies are given for long periods, as they often are, the patient may start to prove the remedy, developing a new set of symptoms. If these remedies are being taken, it is undesirable to continue for longer than three weeks unless the patient is under medical supervision.

CHAPTER ELEVEN

FUTURE DIRECTIONS

Something has gone badly wrong with the health of the western nations. Despite Britain's National Health Service, the incidence of chronic disease in this country, as in other western countries, has risen by leaps and bounds in the last forty years or so, to the extent that such diseases have now reached epidemic proportions, replacing the acute infectious diseases which we had so cleverly vanquished. Similar trends are seen in all the developed countries, and the developing nations are also beginning to follow suit. With all its vast armamentarium of high technology machinery, its sophisticated surgical techniques and its vast array of pharmaceutical drugs, not only is the Health Service unable to stem the tide of disease, it is now beginning to crumble beneath the increasing load of chronic ill-health.

There are several factors which can be identified as possibly being responsible, at least in part, for this sorry state of affairs. These are: increasing environmental pollution; the pharmaceutical approach to treatment – a. drugs, b. immunization schedules; the denial of the spiritual aspects of man.

1. Increasing environmental pollution

This subject was discussed when we considered the diet-based therapies in Chapter 8. The increasing chemicalization of processed foods with a vast array of artificial colouring and flavouring agents, flavour enhancers, texturizers, emulsifiers, preservatives and so on adds a considerable quantity of chemical compounds to our bodies if we eat such products as part or all of our daily diet. Although some manufacturers are now seeing the light and are at last offering products free from most chemical additives, others continue to produce increasingly synthetic items of diet which taste more and more disgusting to the discriminating palate reared on natural produce. This chemical load must have an adverse effect on our bodies because, in the first place, it increases the work which must be done by the body to eliminate it. Kidneys and liver therefore get a heavier work-load.

If the body cannot excrete the chemicals, they have to be stored somewhere. Apart from crystal deposits in joints, gall bladder and kidneys, most of this storage occurs within the body cells, thus increasing the amount of solid material in the cell substance known as the cytoplasm. Most cytoplasmic components are in colloidal solution. Colloids can be in either sol (liquid) or gel (solid) states, and in health a balance is maintained between the two extremes of too sol or too gel. Extra materials stored in the cytoplasm doubtless increase the tendency to the solid (gel) state, thus upsetting the balance within the cells. This in turn will lead to a slowing down of the transport substances within the cells, thus interfering with cellular function. An increasingly solid or gel state of the cells is equated with increasing degeneration in acupuncture terms. Most, if not all, chronic illness is chronic degenerative illness.

This is one side of the food story. The other is the increasing quantities of herbicides, pesticides and fungicides which are used each year in agriculture, horticulture and forestry. These are sprayed with abandon from machines, helicopters and aeroplanes, with very little control over where they land and what else they damage in addition to their intended targets. By their very nature as biocides, that is, life-killers, these things are not readily biodegradable. They therefore tend to build up in the soil and are absorbed by plants grown on that soil. Quantities of herbicides and pesticides over the estimated upper limits of safety are regularly detected in foods eaten in Britain. Again, since these chemicals are designed to be life-killers, their presence in our food is hardly likely to be beneficial.

Both these aspects of food pollution are responsible for a number of cases of chronic ill-health, as can be shown by the improvements which can occur with simple dietary measures alone. They are not, however, the only forms of environmental pollution which assail us. Increasingly we are exposed to petrol exhaust fumes, industrial pollution including acid rain which is currently having such devastating effects on the forests of Scandinavia and Central Europe, radio-active waste and the results of accidents at nuclear power stations and the fluoridation of public water supplies. On the more domestic scene are the aerosol sprays. Many household products come in this form these days: furniture polish, shoe cream, oven-cleaning foam and so on, as well as the traditional air fresheners and hair sprays. The propellants in these sprays contain harmful chemicals including fluoride, which it is impossible to avoid inhaling to some extent or getting in contact with the skin. By their very nature, aerosol sprays get everywhere.

In this context, it is relevant also to mention the widespread use of aluminium cookware and cooking foils. Aluminium became popular for cooking pots and pans because it was cheap. Homoeopathic physicians have long recognized that aluminium can be toxic, especially when heated, and often advise patients with long-standing gastrointestinal problems to avoid using such cookware. A small proportion of patients are very obviously affected by it. Recent suggestions of a link between Alzheimer's disease (one form of senile dementia) and increased levels of aluminium in the brain may just be the tip of an, as yet unrecognized, iceberg.[1]

All in all, the increasing chemicalization of our environment – industrial, agricultural and domestic – probably plays a large part in the increased incidence of chronic degenerative disease. Attention to these aspects may well stem the tide of chronic disease, but it may well not turn it.

2. The pharmaceutical approach to treatment

a. Drugs

Even ten years ago the idea that food additives, pesticides and herbicides could be damaging to health was highly controversial. However, as more information has come to light regarding their effects, more and more people are now recognizing the dangers and seeking ways to avoid them. To suggest, on the other hand, that the orthodox pharmaceutical drugs could be just as harmful is a highly contentious issue but is one which requires serious consideration if we are to turn the tide of chronic disease.

Hahnemann maintained that palliation of the symptoms of disease without actually curing the problem led to suppression of the condition, with its emergence after some time (which could be weeks, months or even years) in an altered and more deep-seated form. He visualized palliation as driving the original problem deeper into the organism, where it continued to grumble away and cause increasingly greater damage.

Most of the modern pharmaceutical drugs simply palliate, they do not really cure. The class names of many of them indicate that they are aimed at specific symptoms –

for instance, anti-inflammatories, anti-depressants, ant-acids, antibiotics. In Hahnemann's terms, such suppression of symptoms could well be expected to be followed by the appearance of more deeply seated problems later on. This, in fact, is the experience of many people on orthodox drugs – that they seem to acquire one problem after another, for which more and more medicines are prescribed, until they are rattling around like a personalized chemist's shop. Not surprisingly they never really feel well, but because they have long since forgotten what it is like to be full of energy, enthusiasm and joy, they accept their lowered state of being as their lot. After all, how often have their doctors told them that they will just have to learn to live with it! And all of this, of course, is in addition to the side-effects which are now a well-recognized feature of most of these drugs.

The suppression of one disease leading to the appearance of another is illustrated by the case of a woman who attended the out-patient department with severe asthma. Many years previously she had developed thyrotoxicosis (overactivity of the thyroid gland) which had been treated with the thyroid-suppressive drug carbimazole. This had been required for only three months and was then discontinued. Six months later she developed asthma, which required frequent admissions to hospital and the use of steroid drugs for many years. Tests showed that she was not allergic to carbimazole.

When the case was retaken from a homoeopathic point of view, the remedy which seemed most appropriate was *Calcarea carbonica* – a form of calcium carbonate prepared from the lining of the oyster shell. Following this, the asthma rapidly cleared up and required no further treatment. Had she been given the calcarea originally, and it is a remedy which contains in its provings many of the symptoms of thyrotoxicosis, it is likely that the asthma would not have developed.

Another case is that of a man who had suffered from eczema for many years. This was treated with steroid creams and after some time he developed asthma. When seen at the clinic, *Arsenicum album* seemed to be the indicated remedy, and this was prescribed. Following this he had a good response and the asthma improved considerably. At a later visit, he was given a higher potency of arsenicum, but this produced a bad aggravation of both the asthma and the eczema which took about two months to settle. Subsequent treatment with the original lower potency finally cleared up firstly the asthma and then the eczema.

Quite apart from their role in suppressing the symptoms of illness, our modern pharmaceutical drugs are synthetic chemicals in a similar class to the food additives which we have already considered. In addition to the pharmacological effects which they have on the body's basic metabolic function, they increase the work which the body has to do in detoxifying and excreting them. It is now recognized that as these functions decrease in older people, so these pharmaceutical drugs have a longer and longer half-life in the body and that doses for elderly people should often be reduced. And again, if the body cannot get rid of them, they add to the increasing piles of junk and debris cluttering up the cells.

Homoeopathic practitioners have for long been aware that lengthy courses of steroid drugs make subsequent homoeopathic treatment of the patient very difficult, if not impossible. The same has been found by the acupuncturists of the Society of Biophysical Medicine who have also observed that heavy courses of antibiotics so alter the electrical characteristics of the body that electrical diagnosis is not possible until several months after the antibiotics have been discontinued.

The orthodox profession itself is currently concerned about the often unthinking way in which antibiotics have been, and still are being, used. Their concern, however, centres mainly on the emergence of increasingly resistant strains of organisms against which the antibiotics become useless. This situation has now developed into a race in which man is barely ahead in the production of new and more effective antibiotics, with the resistant organisms hard on his heels. For how much longer can we keep ahead?

The concern of the alternative medical scene includes this aspect of the antibiotics but goes much further. The alternative practitioners feel that antibiotic therapy, although it is directed against the infecting organisms and not the patient, is still a form of suppressive therapy and wonder what long-term effects it might have on the whole of the sensitive, delicately balanced immune system. Since the immune system is our defence mechanism against harmful environmental agents – be they infections, toxins or stresses of various kinds – widespread upset in this area could be catastrophic. Some years ago, an eminent homoeopathic prescriber predicted that we were laying ourselves open to invasion by as yet unknown diseases against which we would have little defence. The appearance recently of Legionnaire's Disease and AIDS would seem to vindicate his opinion.

That antibiotics can affect the immune system is borne out by the allergies which some patients develop to certain antibiotics, particularly those of the penicillin group. A man of forty who sustained an injury was given injections of penicillin and tetanus toxoid. A few days later he developed swelling of the ankles and knees which continued for two weeks and would not settle until he was given a homoeopathic preparation of penicillin which cleared up the problem.

b. Immunization schedules

It is not only the widespread use of pharmaceutical drugs and antibiotics, however, which causes concern to some members of the medical profession. One of the major triumphs of the twentieth century has been the virtual elimination, in the developed countries, of the great infectious epidemics which used to ravage our populations. This has been achieved largely by a combination of improved public health – principally good sanitation and safe water supplies – and the vaccination programmes.

Vaccination really started in Britain with Jenner's experiments in preventing smallpox by infecting instead with cowpox. Interestingly, Jenner's first experiment was conducted in 1796, the same year that Hahnemann published his first article on the idea of treatment by similars. With increasing knowledge of antibodies and how they work, the idea of vaccination was rapidly developed in the twentieth century to produce safe vaccination programmes for all the acute infectious diseases. Complicated vaccination schedules now exist whereby small children, starting at about four to six months of age, are protected against measles, whooping cough, diphtheria, tetanus and polio, with tuberculosis vaccination often introduced later. Not so many years ago when a baby was born in hospital, it was difficult *not* to have him or her immunized against tuberculosis before being allowed home!

Quite apart from adverse side-effects, principally in the form of brain damage, which can arise particularly from whooping cough and measles vaccinations, and which is itself another highly contentious issue at the present time, there is another worry about these large-scale vaccination programmes. Many of them start at an early age – before six months – at a time when the developing immune system has not yet matured. Also, in an attempt to minimize the trauma to a small child, such things as the triple vaccine (a combination of diphtheria, tetanus and whooping cough – all in the one injection) have been developed. The baby's immune system is thus being bombarded by these antigens at an age when under natural conditions this would not normally happen, since breast-fed babies obtain a passive immunity from their mothers which protects them up to, and often beyond, six months of age, by which time their own immune system has matured. In addition, they are often bombarded with several antigens at a time – again a situation which seldom occurs naturally. What effect this has on the subsequent harmonious functioning of the immune system is difficult to assess. What is apparent, though, is the ever-increasing incidence of allergy in the population – to the extent that now about one child in four is allergic to something. Allergy is defined as a state of abnormal functioning of the immune system. Whether the widespread use of immunization schedules plays a part in the increasing allergic state of the nation or not is still debatable, but is certainly well worth bearing in mind.

Another aspect of immune system dysfunction is the area of the auto-immune diseases in which the body ceases to recognize its own tissues, treats them as foreign and so proceeds to destroy them. Whether the increased incidence of auto-immune disease is also related in any way to the vaccination programmes is as yet quite unknown.

3. The denial of the spiritual aspects of man

This is a totally different subject from the two already discussed and is involved with the more subtle factors concerned in the production of disease. If we consider ourselves to be purely material beings with a finite existence in this world, at the end of which we cease to exist and that is that, then life becomes meaningless. Not so much when we are young, and all the challenge of life is still before us, but once we have achieved a reasonable level of material comfort, the question arises, what next? And if, when we die, there is nothing more, then what is the point of striving to achieve anything at all, apart from the purely material pleasures? As the years pass, the outlook becomes increasingly meaningless and bleak, empty and frustrating. Since all levels of the organism interweave, interact and affect each other, this must have repercussions on the mental and emotional levels, and it would not be surprising if physical symptoms did not also, finally, appear.

The increasingly material, mechanistic view of the world is doubtless responsible for many of the frustrations, anxieties, disturbed sleep patterns and subtle mental/emotional imbalances that many people suffer from these days. If we have no sense of our true identity we are adrift in the world, at the mercy of all it cares to throw at us, and in control of nothing, least of all ourselves. In the opinion of one of our Dutch colleagues, a disordered sense of 'I am', and blocks in our ability to contact our own divine souls, are at the root of many cases of cancer seen today. Such patients will never be cured by drugs, radiotherapy, diet therapy, vitamins or homoeopathy. They can only be truly helped if they are able to re-establish their connections with their inner being, their divine soul, and in so doing recognize that the material world is *not* all that there is. With such a realization comes a new meaning for life. It is no longer seen as the pointless grind that formerly it appeared to be. New dimensions of being, health and joy come within one's grasp.

So here we are towards the end of the twentieth century, a nation maimed and wounded in its health. An increasing burden of chronic ill-health overwhelms us and orthodox approaches appear to be incapable of stemming the tide, let alone turning it.

Hahnemann considered that chronic disease was tied up with what he called the 'inherited miasms' – a view since validated by genetics, which recognizes that chronic disease is the resultant of internal, inherited, genetic factors and the external adverse environmental influences. Hahnemann believed that the effects of infections and toxins in one generation could be passed on to successive generations, and the discovery that viruses can indeed insert themselves into our genetic material (the DNA) has lent much credence to his view. He developed a series of remedies which he called nosodes, prepared from specific disease products, which he used as specific antidotes to these diseases in a way similar to the antibodies with which we are now all familiar. These nosodes can be used to counteract the inherited traits lying at the root of many chronic conditions.

A recent development of the homoeopathic concept is the field of psionic medicine.[2] Over the past thirty years George Laurence[3] has devised and developed a method of studying the changes which occur in basic body protein during illness. This is done using dowsing techniques which make it possible to detect changes occurring at the DNA/RNA level when the individual is exposed to the influences of toxic factors – the object being to determine *why* rather than just *that* a person is ill.

These factors may be acquired during the lifetime of the person or inherited (Hahnemann's miasms). Apart from their effects on DNA or RNA, the influence of these toxins on systems, organs, tissues and even fluids in the body can be measured, confirming the history given by the patient. Once the composition of the toxic load has been determined, the order in which the toxic factors should be eliminated, using single or perhaps complex remedies, can be worked out – the remedies being selected specifically in relation to the toxic factors involved in the condition. The potency of each remedy and the frequency and duration of dosage can also be measured precisely. Where complex remedies are used, each component must be in its own correct potency and these potencies are virtually always in the range 6X to 12C.

Of great interest here is the observation that certain patterns of toxic factors are associated with particular presentations of illness and this gives greater meaning to family histories both prospectively and retrospectively. One can begin to see where certain tendencies have arisen, and the elimination of inherited and heritable toxins means sparing the next generations from these toxins and, therefore, from their effects.

With psionic medicine, therefore, the patient's problems are cleared layer by layer, rather like peeling an onion. As each layer is removed, another deeper layer usually emerges, thus initiating the opposite process to that obtained with suppressive, palliative drugs. Of course homoeopathic practitioners can select remedies and nosodes to clear toxins and miasms without the help of the psionic approach. There is, however, often much argument as to the order in which homoeopathic remedies should be given and even, in some schools, as to whether the patient really needs more than one remedy. As we saw in Chapter 6 some schools of thought, particularly in South America, consider that all aspects of a case can be viewed as various expressions of just one remedy and that the patient does not change his or her remedy at all throughout life. Such views, however, are not generally accepted in Britain.

The advantage of the psionic approach is that at the end of the patient's analysis, the prescription with the remedies in the order in which they are to be given has been derived. It is the experience of psionic practitioners that in chronic cases several remedies are always required as several toxic factors need to be eliminated. The situation at the end of the course of treatment should be that all the inherited and acquired toxic influences have been cleared. While this may not have a significant effect on the patient's own health and function, if much irreversible damage has already been done, it holds out the opportunity of reducing the genetic load. Therefore if patients are treated before they start a family, their children should be free of inherited miasms, thus reducing their susceptibility to chronic diseases.

Another field which has attracted a number of investigators in the present century is that of bio-electric medicine, a concept which has intimate connections with homoeopathy. In Chapter 4 it was shown how all chemical and biochemical reactions are essentially rearrangements of electrical fields of force; the electrical charges being properties of the sub-atomic particles from which all physical matter is created, whether chemical or biological. All living creatures are highly complex electrical systems – a concept known to the ancient Chinese acupuncturists but not appreciated in the west until the beginning of the present century.

Dr Starr White of Los Angeles is credited with being the first person in the west to notice a relationship between a human subject and his orientation with respect to the earth's magnetic field. Normally if one percusses the abdomen of a person, a resonant note is obtained due to air in the intestines. Starr White noticed that if a subject whose abdomen he was percussing turned so that he was standing aligned at right angles to the earth's magnetic field, areas of dullness could be detected which were not present if the subject were standing parallel to the earth's magnetic field.

Dr Abrams of San Fancisco repeated Starr White's findings and investigated them further. He found that patients with cancer had areas of dullness near the navel and patients with tuberculosis had a dull area below the navel. Abrams was able to map out areas of the abdomen which reacted to different diseases, some of which overlapped. He considered that he was dealing with an electrical phenomenon and that it should be possible to design a machine which could measure the changes obtained in electrical terms. To this end he built a box containing a series of variable resistors and using this instrument he found that he could distinguish one disease from another using ohms (the measurement of resistance) as his measurement parameter. He found that each disease seemed to be related to a particular degree of resistance to the electrical flow, so that it could be expressed numerically in terms of a certain number of ohms.

Abrams further discovered that if he inserted a blood spot from the patient into his circuit, it would act as a witness for the patient who was then substituted for by a normal healthy subject whose abdomen was percussed. This meant that patients living at a distance from Dr Abrams did not need to travel to San Francisco to be diagnosed by him, but could send a blood sample from which the diagnosis could be made.

Dr W. E. Boyd in Glasgow[1] also studied this phenomenon of changes in abdominal percussion note under certain conditions. He was of the opinion that he was dealing with something akin to a radio signal rather than an electrical signal as Abrams believed. To study this, he designed and built his emanometer which screened the subject whose abdomen was percussed from all environmental electro-magnetic waves, as well as from the operator and the blood spot, or whatever other substances were used in the circuit. Using this instrument, Boyd was able to select the appropriate homoeopathic treatment. This he was able to demonstrate successfully, and with a high degree of statistical significance, to the Horder committee, a well-qualified group of two doctors and three scientists under the leadership of Lord Horder, which was set up in 1924 to investigate his claims. The Horder committee had no option but to admit that the emanometer was capable of demonstrating a genuine phenomenon, that of an electrical field both around the human body and homoeopathic remedies.

Using the emanometer for his remedy selection, Boyd found himself becoming closer to Hahnemann in his methods of prescribing, giving one remedy and waiting perhaps two to three months before either repeating or changing it. The emanometer, however, was cumbersome and difficult to use, and Boyd found that it was impossible to dispense with the healthy subject. The instrument, therefore, was not widely used by other practitioners.

Further advances in electrical approaches to diagnosis were made by the German doctor Reinholdt Voll in the early 1950s. Being trained in both homoeopathy and acupuncture, Voll thought that it should be possible to measure the electrical resistance of acupuncture points and found that this was indeed so. From these observations he went on to lay the foundations of electro-acupuncture, a technique which is much in favour at the moment in the treatment of many conditions including drug addiction. Voll also wondered if there might be a relationship between an acupuncture meridian and the organ associated with it by the ancient Chinese acupuncturists, and he was able to demonstrate that the meridians did bear some relationship to the organ after which they were named. Using electrical circuitry, he was able to demonstrate that if a meridian was not functioning correctly, he could detect a drop in voltage on specific points located on that meridian. This he called an indicator drop. He then found that if he incorporated homoeopathic remedies into his machine in series with the patient and the measurement probe, the readings on the meridian returned to normal when the appropriate remedy was introduced into the circuit. This concept is essentially similar to that of Boyd's emanometer, but the apparatus was much simpler and easier to use.

Although Voll's technique was found to be thera-
peutically effective it, too, was laborious and time-
consuming. Dr Helmut Schimmel, one of Voll's pupils,
simplified the system by using witnesses of each organ –
that is, preparations of the tissues of that organ – instead of
measuring points on each meridian in turn. Schimmel used
just one point, either on a finger or a toe, and used the
witnesses of the various organs to assess whether they were
normal or not. When an abnormality was found, it was
corrected by incorporating remedies in series, as had been
done by Voll. This technique is quicker, easier and more
reliable than Voll's original method and is the origin of the
Vegatest machine which is now used by a number of
practitioners both on the continent and in Britain, and is
basic to the recently developed discipline of bio-electronic
regulatory (BER) medicine.[5] The Vegatest machine can be
used to identify unsuspected precipitating factors and
causes in disease such as infected foci, toxins and inherited
factors, and can also be used as an aid to homoeopathic
remedy selection.

The above methods are dependent, to a certain extent,
on the trained reactions of the operator and include an
unavoidable subjective element. A more objective approach
is that of the segmental electrogram which detects areas of
electrical imbalance or disturbance in different segments of
the body. The patient's history and a clinical examination
can then help in identifying which organs within that
segment are under stress or are diseased. This technique
often detects electrical imbalances prior to pathological
changes actually occurring, and the imbalances so detected
have been shown to return to a more normal pattern following appropriate treatment.

Another approach to the electrical aspects of the body is
that developed by Eeman around the 1920s.[6] He looked on

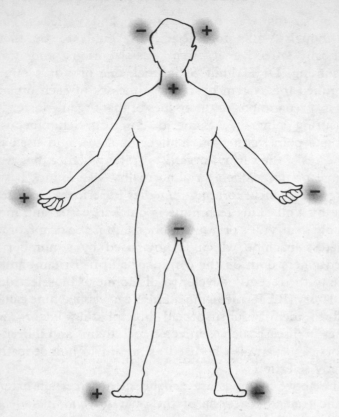

Figure 12. Classical diagram of human polarities

the body as a sort of battery with positive and negative areas as shown in Figure 12. He experimented with connecting up the positive and negative areas with copper wires and grids as shown in Figure 13 and found that such a circuit had a very relaxing effect on any subject placed in it. Crossing the legs produced an even more profound state of relaxation, an observation used in some meditation techniques. Eeman then conceived the idea of connecting two subjects in series, positive to negative, and found that if they were trained to relax properly, they would often fall

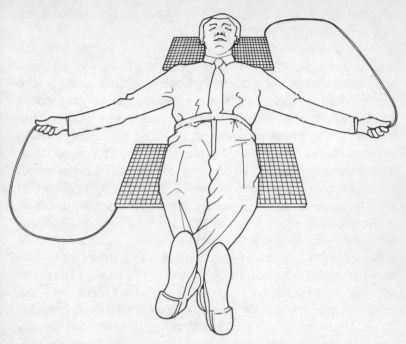

Figure 13. One subject in relaxation circuit, showing copper gauze mats and wire connections

asleep and awake simultaneously. After a number of experiments he concluded that there was probably some sort of energy flowing through the wire which would synchronize the two individuals in the circuit. Moreover, he found that if he connected them positive to positive and negative to negative, then instead of becoming relaxed they became restless, anxious and irritable. He was able to repeat these observations consistently using a hidden switch so that he could change the circuitry unknown to the two subjects. He could therefore put them into a state of relaxation or a state of irritability literally at the flick of a switch. Eeman also found that if he put crude drugs such as aspirin into the circuit, the subject would experience the effects of taking a large dose of aspirin. The same thing could be done for any drug.

We ourselves have adapted this idea of Eeman's to the use of homoeopathic potencies. Using the Eeman circuits, we found that by introducing a homoeopathic potency into the circuit in series with the subject, the subject could experience the symptoms and signs of the remedy within minutes of it being introduced, and the experiment could be continued for as long as the subject felt comfortable. Not everyone is sensitive to every remedy, of course; we all have our individual sensitivities. This technique, however, can be used as a rapid screening method to find which individuals are sensitive to which remedies. Individuals who are found in this way to be sensitive to various remedies can be invited to take part in confirmatory provings of that remedy if this is required, either using the Eeman circuit or by the traditional method whereby volunteers take the remedy in question daily for a period of several weeks. With the Eeman circuit, many symptoms of the remedy can be experienced within a matter of an hour or less, which makes this technique much less laborious and much more rapid and efficient than the traditional method. The Eeman circuitry also has applications as a therapeutic tool and this aspect is currently being investigated.

Another piece of modern wizardry which is not un-connected with the subject under discussion is the Kirlian camera. Kirlian photography was developed in Russia by a husband-and-wife team named Kirlian and it records on photographic paper or plates the electrical fields sur-rounding the bodies of living things – plants, animals or human beings. It is used by some acupuncturists of the Biophysical Medicine Society to visualize the electrical state of the acupuncture meridians, showing whether they are normal, over-active or under-active electrically. In this context it is used in a similar way to the Voll and Vegatest methods to diagnose electrical imbalances in the body. It is claimed that Kirlian photography can pick up electrical fields around homoeopathic remedies as well as around living beings – a claim in line with W. E. Boyd's observations with his emanometer of an electrical field not only around his human subjects but around homoeopathic remedies as well. The full potential of Kirlian photography in diagnosis and remedy selection remains to be explored.

The twentieth century has therefore seen an increasing interest in the electrical aspects of the body and a fuller appreciation of the fact that we are all, at heart, complex electrical fields. Using electrical instrumentation it has proved possible to detect and correct electrical imbalances before obvious physical changes – in medical terms, gross pathology – occur. The implication of this is that the roots of disease lie in electrical imbalances at a more subtle level of organization than the physical. The sequence of events can be visualized as an electrical imbalance which leads to a biochemical imbalance, which leads in turn to problems within individual cells and finally to obvious physical changes of the kind that can be detected on routine clinical examination. If we go back to the diagram in Chapter 4 (Figure 5) of the increasing levels of organization from the sub-atomic particle to the individual living being, we can appreciate better the full implications.

Using the electrical methods of diagnosis, imbalances can be detected at the level of the atoms and sub-atomic particles. If these can be corrected before they impinge on the molecules then imbalances at the biochemical level, and all the levels subsequent to it, will be avoided – an efficient form of preventive medicine. Obviously, the earlier in the chain of events the abnormality can be treated, the easier it is to effect a cure.

The use of subtle methods of remedy selection to prescribe the correct homoeopathic remedy even before the full symptom picture develops, or techniques such as electro-acupuncture to correct, directly, the electrical imbalances, offers unparalleled opportunities for disease prevention and treatment.

We know that some people are markedly affected by thunder and that others feel achy in wet weather. Such weather modalities are familiar to homoeopathic prescribers and are an integral part of some remedy pictures. Certain winds such as the föhn in Switzerland, the mistral in the South of France, the sirocco in Italy and the sharav in Israel, which bring with them an excess of positive atmospheric ions, make some people feel ill, liable to infections or even murderous or suicidal. Accident, murder and suicide rates are frequently higher at times when such winds are blowing.

Then there is the 'sick building syndrome' – modern buildings with ducted air central-heating systems and air-conditioning in which the lighting is of the fluorescent variety, and which are often associated with a much higher incidence of occupational ill-health than traditional buildings without ducted air systems and with normal incandescent rather than fluorescent lighting. The increased use of video screens in many occupations is another potential hazard.

We have now, however, in these developing techniques of electrical diagnosis, potential tools for assessing the effects of ionization and electro-magnetic waves on our bodies and on the environment as a whole. Looking back over this chapter, we can suggest a number of ways in which medicine can begin to stem, and turn back, the tide of ill-health both in this country and abroad.

• In the first place attention should be given to reducing pollution and to the provision of a natural, healthy, pollution-free diet. Chemical products which could be detrimental to health and the environment as a whole should be phased out, or safe alternatives sought.

● Second, the methods of treatment should be reconsidered. Suppressive therapies should be avoided wherever possible and more attention paid to the safer alternatives such as homoeopathy, acupuncture and the other alternative approaches.

● Third, more attention should be given to the whole being of man. A swing away from a grossly materialistic outlook would be beneficial to our total health and well-being, which involves far more than purely material needs. This trend has been gaining momentum in the past decade or so with the increasing interest in yoga and other meditation and spiritual techniques such as transcendental meditation, mind control, the charismatic movement, Subud[7] and so on. If we are to be truly healthy, we have to have meaning in our lives.

● Finally, the development of psionic medicine – an extension of homoeopathy – and the bio-electrical diagnostic methods offer precise and measurable ways into the clearing of the inherited predispositions, or miasms, and the subtle electrical imbalances. The implications of a widespread application of these approaches are exciting, since they offer an opportunity for treating many conditions which are, at present, considered incurable. Whether they have the power to cure the more obviously inherited genetic diseases and inborn errors is a challenging field for future research.

REFERENCES AND NOTES

CHAPTER ONE. Homoeopathy in Action

1. All homoeopathic remedies are named in Latin. It was the language of science in Hahnemann's day (see p.71) and still is in some disciplines, for example, botany and zoology. Remedies of plant and animal origin are named after the species and remedies of mineral origin bear the Latinized version of the chemical name – for example, common salt (sodium chloride) is *Natrum muriaticum*, white arsenic is *Arsenicum album*, silver nitrate is *Argentum nitricum* and so on.

CHAPTER THREE. Ways in Which Doctors Come into Homoeopathy

1. Dowsing is a method of obtaining information which is not normally accessible to the mind. The best-known form is water-divining, where the practitioner uses rods of various types (traditionally a forked hazel twig) to detect the presence of water under the ground. It is possible to dowse for almost anything and commercially this faculty is used to detect not only water and the lines of water and sewage pipes, but also oil and mineral deposits. It can also be used to locate lost items and to detect buried objects at archaeological sites. In a medical context it can be helpful in diagnosing what is wrong with a patient and in selecting an appropriate remedy. In these latter instances a pendulum – rather than a rod or twig – is normally used.

2. Radionics is a discipline in which the patient's problem is diagnosed using a dowsing technique often with the help of a radionic diagnostic machine. The treatment is also found by dowsing and the appropriate remedy can then be 'broadcast' to the patient, again using the radionic machine. For fuller details those interested may like to read *Report on Radionics* by Edward W. Russell (2nd edition, Neville Spearman, 1979).

3. Deoxyribonucleic acid (DNA) is the name given in biochemistry to the complex biological material which is responsible for passing on the inherited traits from one generation to the next. The unit of DNA responsible for each inherited characteristic is known as a gene and the effects of many genes are involved in the transmission of even simple characteristics like height, body build or eye colour. The genes are grouped together to form structures called chromosomes which are located in the nucleus of the cell. Apart from the reproductive cells (the

sperm and the ova) each cell in the body should have an identical chromosome complement.

4. Ribonucleic acid (RNA) is the name given biochemically to a complex biological molecule similar to, but not identical with, DNA. The function of RNA is to act as an intermediary between the gene (the unit of inheritance) and protein formation, which is the first step in utilizing the information carried in the gene and transforming it into physical characteristics.

CHAPTER FOUR. Background of Health and Disease

1. Vithoulkas, George, *The Science of Homoeopathy*, A.S.O.H.M., 1978.

2. Watson, E. Grant, *The Mystery of Physical Life*, Abelard-Schuman, London, New York, Toronto, 1964.

3. Cantle, S., 'Consultant Stands by Finger Regrowth Claim', *Hospital Doctor*, 15 September 1983, p. 28.

CHAPTER SEVEN. How Does Homoeopathy Work?

1. Stillinger, F. H., 'Water Revisited', *Science*, *209*, 1980, pp. 451–7.

2. Narten, A. H. and Levy, H. A., 'Observed Diffraction Pattern and Proposed Models for Liquid Water', *Science*, *165*, 1969, pp. 447–54.

3. Frank, H. S., 'The Structure of Ordinary Water', *Science*, *169*, 1970, pp. 635–41.

4. Eisenberg, D. and Kauzmann, W., *The Structure and Properties of Water*, Clarendon Press, 1969.

5. Barnard, G. P. and Stephenson, J. H., 'Microdose Paradox: A New Biophysical Concept', *J. Am. Inst. Hom.*, *60*, 1967, pp. 277–86.

6. Heintz, E., 'The Physical Effect of Highly Diluted Potentized Substances', *Die Naturwissenschaften*, *29*, 1941, pp. 713–25.

7. Smith, R. B. and Boericke, G. W., 'Modern Instrumentation for the Evaluation of Homoeopathic Drug Structure', *J. Am. Inst. Hom.*, *59*, 1966, pp. 263–80.

8. Wolfram, S., 'Cellular Automata as Models of Complexity', *Nature*, *311*, 1984, pp. 419–24.

9. Horrobin, D. F., *Prostaglandins: Physiology, Pharmacology and Clinical Significance*, Churchill Livingstone, Edinburgh, 1978.

10. Hahnemann, S., *The Chronic Diseases: Their Peculiar Nature and their Homoeopathic Cure*, C. Ringer and Co., Calcutta, translation of 2nd edition, 1835.

CHAPTER EIGHT. The Relationship of Homoeopathy to Other Therapies

1. Enzymes and co-enzymes: an enzyme is a specialized protein which allows a living organism to carry out complex chemical reactions at body temperature and normal atmospheric pressure. Usually each specific reaction has its own enzyme although occasionally an enzyme may be involved in two or more closely similar reactions. Many enzymes require substances called co-factors or co-enzymes to help them work. These are small molecules (often vitamins or trace elements) and this is the reason why these substances are so essential.

2. Diesendorf, M., 'The Mystery of Declining Tooth Decay', *Nature*, *322*, 1986, pp. 125–9.

3. Smith, G. E., 'A Surfeit of Fluoride?', *Sci. Prog. Oxf.*, *69*, 1985, pp. 429–42.

4. The term saturated, as applied to fats, refers to the number of hydrogen atoms associated with each carbon atom in the molecule. The backbone of the fatty acid chain is composed of a number of carbon atoms linked to hydrogen atoms thus:

$$\begin{array}{ccccccc} & H & H & H & H & \\ & | & | & | & | & \\ H- & C- & C- & C- & C- & \text{etc.} \\ & | & | & | & | & \\ & H & H & H & H & \end{array}$$

Each carbon atom has four bonds or valencies. In the main part of the chain, two of these are attached to other carbon atoms and two are attached to hydrogen atoms as shown above. This gives a saturated fat which is solid at room temperature.

Sometimes, however, not all the spare bonds are taken up with hydrogen atoms, giving a situation like this:

$$\begin{array}{ccccccc} & H & H & H & H & \\ & | & | & | & | & \\ H- & C- & C & = & C- & C- & \text{etc.} \\ & | & & & | & \\ & H & & & H & \end{array}$$

In this case, two of the carbon atoms each have one hydrogen atom less than they could have, and therefore have an extra bond to each other. This gives rise to what is called, in chemistry, a double bond. Such a fat is unsaturated, that is, it can take up more hydrogen to become saturated. The vegetable oils are polyunsaturated which means that they contain several double bonds, which makes them liquid at room temperature.

A fully saturated molecule is symmetrical and can only have one configuration. An unsaturated molecule is not symmetrical. The example shown above can have two possible configurations known as cis (hydrogens on the same side of the double bond) and trans (hydrogens on opposite sides). These derive from the Latin *cis* (this side) and *trans* (across), as in Cis-Alpine and Trans-Alpine Gaul in Roman times.

cis form   trans form

The cis form is the one favoured by nature.

5. Barlow, W., *The Alexander Principle*, Arrow Books, 1975.

6. Chancellor, Phillip M., *Handbook of the Bach Flower Remedies*, C. W. Daniel Ltd, Ashingdon, Essex, 1971.

7. Dosch, Peter, *Manual of Neural Therapy According to Huneke* (English edition), Haug Verlag, Heidelberg, 1984.

8. Autogenic training is a technique similar to autohypnosis which is used to achieve inner calm and relaxation. It incorporates aspects of hypnosis, psychoanalysis and yoga and can be a valuable aid in improving one's performance in whatever skill requires perfecting. It is often used by skiers, tennis players and participants in other sports but can be applied in any situation where performance requires improvement.

9. Autohypnosis is a form of hypnosis in which the patient is his own hypnotist. He is taught by the therapist to put himself into a state of deep relaxation in which he is open to positive suggestions which he makes to himself for improving his well-being, his self-image, his ability to cope with difficult situations and so on. This technique makes the patient independent of the therapist and gives him a tool which he can use whenever the need arises.

10. Blyth, Peter, lecture on hypnotherapy, Glasgow, 1986.

11. Gibson, S. L. M., 'Arthritis', *Homoeopathy Today*, autumn issue, 1985, pp. 22–5.

12. Gibson, R. G., Gibson, S. L. M., Conway, V. and Chappell, D., '*Perna canaliculus* in the Treatment of Arthritis', *Practitioner, 224*, 1980, pp. 955–60.

CHAPTER NINE. Does Homoeopathy Work? The Results of Research

1. Narten, A. H. and Levy, H. A., 'Observed Diffraction Pattern and Proposed Models of Liquid Water', *Science*, *165*, 1969, pp. 447–54.

2. Symons, M. C. R., Blandamer, M. J. and Fox, M. F., 'Is Water Kinky?', *New Scientist*, *34*, 1967, pp. 345–6.

3. Stillinger, F. H., 'Water Revisited', *Science*, *209*, 1980, pp. 451–7.

4. Frank, H. S., 'The Structure of Ordinary Water', *Science*, *169*, 1970, pp. 635–41.

5. Schwenk, Theodor, *Sensitive Chaos*, Rudolf Steiner Press, 1965.

6. Bridgman, P. W., *The Physics of High Pressure*, Bell, 1949.

7. Barnard, G. P., 'Microdose Paradox: A New Concept', *J. Am. Inst. Hom.*, *58*, 1965, pp. 205–12.

8. Barnard, G. P. and Stephenson, J. H., 'Microdose Paradox: A New Biophysical Concept', *J. Am. Inst. Hom.*, *60*, 1967, pp. 277–86.

9. Stillinger, F. H., 'Water Revisited', *Science*, *209*, 1980, pp. 451–7.

10. Anbar, M., 'Chemical Reactions Induced by Sound', *New Scientist*, *30*, 1966, pp. 365–7.

11. Heintz, E., 'The Physical Effect of Highly Diluted, Potentized Substances', *Die Naturwissenschaften*, *29*, 1941, pp. 713–25.

12. Smith, R. B. and Boericke, G. W., 'Modern Instrumentation for the Evaluation of Homoeopathic Drug Structure', *J. Am. Inst. Hom.*, *59*, 1966, pp. 263–80.

13. Kolisko, L., *Physical and Physiological Demonstration of the Effect of the Smallest Entities 1923–1959*, Arbeitsgemeinschaft anthrop. Arzte, Stuttgart, 1959.

14. Boyd, W. E., 'Biochemical and Biological Evidence of the Activity of High Potencies', *Br. Hom. J.*, *44*, 1954, pp. 6–44.

15. Basold, A., *Elem. Naturwiss.*, *8*, 1968, p. 32.

16. Bockemuhl, J., *Elem. Naturwiss.*, *8*, 1968, p. 27.

17. Flemming, H., *Elem. Naturwiss.*, *20*, 1974, p. 26.

18. Amons, F. and Mansvelt, J., *Elem. Naturwiss.*, *17*, 1972, p. 27.

19. Amons, F. and Mansvelt, J., *Zeitschrift Naturforsch.*, *30*, 1975, p. 613.

20. Kollerstrom, J., 'Basic Scientific Research into the "Low-Dose Effect"', *Br. Hom. J.*, *71*, 1982, pp. 41–7.

21. Boiron, J. and Marin, M., 'Action d'une 15e CH de sulfate de cuivre sur la culture de Chlorella vulgaris', *Assises scientifiques homéopathiques*, 9, 1970, pp. 25–32.

22. Graviou, E. and Biron, A., *Les annales homéopathiques françaises*, 13, 1971, pp. 539–48.

23. Moss, V. A., Roberts, J. A. and Simpson, H. K. L., 'The Effect of Copper Sulphate on the Growth of the Alga Chlorella', *Br. Hom. J.*, 66, 1977, pp. 169–77.

24. Moss, V. A., Roberts, J. A. and Simpson, K., 'The Action of "Low Potency" Homoeopathic Remedies on the Movement of Guinea-Pig Macrophages and Human Leucocytes', *Br. Hom. J.*, 71, 1982, pp. 48–61.

25. Pelikan, W. and Unger, G., 'The Activity of Potentized Substances', *Br. Hom. J.*, 60, 1971, pp. 233–66.

26. Jones, R. L. and Jenkins, M. D., 'Plant Responses to Homoeopathic Remedies', *Br. Hom. J.*, 70, 1981, pp. 120–28.

27. Jones, R. L. and Jenkins, M. D., 'Comparison of Wheat and Yeast as *in vitro* Models for Investigating Homoeopathic Medicines', *Br. Hom. J.*, 72, 1983, pp. 143–7.

28. Jones, R. L. and Jenkins, M. D., 'Effects of Hand and Machine Succussion on *in vitro* Activity of Potencies of Pulsatilla', *Br. Hom. J.*, 72, 1983, pp. 217–23.

29. Steffen, W., 'Growth of Yeast Cultures as *in vitro* Model for Investigating Homoeopathic Medicines: Some Further Studies', *Br. Hom. J.*, 74, 1985, pp. 132–9.

30. Singh, L. M. and Gupta, G., 'Antiviral Efficacy of Homoeopathic Drugs against Animal Viruses', *Br. Hom. J.*, 74, 1985, pp. 168–74.

31. Lapp, C., Wurmser, L. and Ney, J., 'Mobilisation de l'arsenic fixe chez le cobaye sous l'influence de doses infinitésimales d'arséniate de sodium', *Thérapie*, 10, 1955, pp. 625–38.

32. Boiron, J., Abecassis, J. and Belon, P., 'A Pharmacological Study of the Retention and Mobilization of Arsenic as Caused by Hahnemannian Potencies of *Arsenicum album*', *Aspects of Research in Homoeopathy*, 1, 1983, pp. 19–25.

33. Boiron, J., Abecassis, J. and Belon, P., 'The Effects of Hahnemannian *Mercurius corrosivus* Potencies upon the Multiplication of Cultured Fibroblasts Poisoned with Mercury Chloride, ibid., pp. 51–60.

34. Boiron, J., Abecassis, J. and Belon, P., 'The Action of *Gelsemium sempervirens* Tincture upon the Capture of Neurotransmitters by Synaptosomal Preparations of Various Fractions of Rat Brain', ibid., pp. 39–50.

35. Boiron, J., Abecassis, J. and Belon, P., 'The Effects of Hahnemannian Potencies of 7C Histaminum and 7C *Apis mellifica* upon Basophil Degranulation in Allergic Patients', ibid., pp. 61–6.

36. Gibson, R. G. and Gibson, S. L. M., 'A New Aspect of Psora: The Recognition and Treatment of House-Dust-Mite Allergy', *Br. Hom. J.*, 69, 1980, pp. 151–8.

37. Reilly, D. T. and Taylor, M. A., 'Potent Placebo or Potency?', *Br. Hom. J.*, 74, 1985, pp. 65–75.

38. Reilly, D. T., Taylor, M. A., McSharry, C. and Aitchison, T., 'Is Homoeopathy a Placebo Response', *Lancet, ii*, 1986, pp. 881–6.

39. Gibson, R. G., Gibson, S. L. M., MacNeill, A. D., Gray, G. H., Dick, W. C. and Buchanan, W. W., 'Salicylates and Homoeopathy in Rheumatoid Arthritis: Preliminary Observations', *Br. J. Clin. Pharmac.*, 6, 1978, pp. 391–5.

40. Gibson, R. G., Gibson, S. L. M., MacNeill, A. D. and Buchanan, W. W., 'Homoeopathic Therapy in Rheumatoid Arthritis: Evaluation by Double-Blind Clinical Therapeutic Trial', *Br. J. Clin. Pharmac.*, 9, 1980, pp. 453–9.

41. Gibson, R. G., Gibson, S. L. M., MacNeill, A. D. and Buchanan, W. W., 'The Place for Non-Pharmaceutical Therapy in Chronic Rheumatoid Arthritis: A Critical Study of Homoeopathy', *Br. Hom. J.*, 69, 1980, pp. 121–33.

42. Shipley, M., Berry, H., Broster, G., Jenkins, M., Clover, A. and Williams, I., 'Controlled Trial of Homoeopathic Treatment of Arthritis', *Lancet, i*, 1983, pp. 97–8.

43. Gracely, R. H., Dubner, R., Deeter, W. R. and Wolskee, P. J., 'Clinicians' Expectations Influence Placebo Analgesia', *Lancet, i*, 1985, p. 43.

CHAPTER ELEVEN. Future Directions

1. Candy, J. M. *et al.*, 'Aluminosilicates and Senile Plaque Formation in Alzheimer's Disease, *Lancet, i*, 1986, pp. 354–7.

2. Reyner, J. H., *Psionic Medicine: The Study and Treatment of the Causative Factors in Illness*, Routledge & Kegan Paul, 1974, 1982.

3. Laurence, George, 'The Unitary Conception of Disease in Relation to Radiesthesia and Homoeopathy', *Radiesthesia*, *iv*, 1952, pp. 68–79.

4. Boyd, W. E., 'Electro-Medical Research and Homoeopathy', *Br. Hom. J.*, *20*, 1930, pp. 299–317.

5. Kenyon, Julian N., *21st-Century Medicine: A Layman's Guide to the Medicine of the Future*, Thorsons Publishers Limited, Wellingborough, 1986.

6. Eeman, L. E., *Co-operative Healing*, Frederick Muller, 1947.

7. Subud is a spiritual brotherhood which originated in Indonesia in the 1920s. It is not, in itself, a religion but embraces all religions, recognizing the validity of each. It has no religious dogma or teaching and is open to all who are willing to surrender themselves to the will of God. The name Subud is an abbreviation of three words of Sanskrit origin: susila, budhi and dharma. Susila implies human behaviour in accordance with the will of God, budhi is the inner force or life force in all creatures, including man, which draws them towards God, and dharma implies sincere surrender and submission to the will of God. The aim of Subud is to enhance our well-being, that of our fellow human beings and of the world at large, and to make our planet a better, saner and more harmonious place in which to live. This can only be achieved through submitting to, and living in harmony with, the will of God.

Appendix 1 Useful Home Remedies

Although the homoeopathic treatment of chronic illness is difficult and should always be carried out by a homoeopathic practitioner, injuries and acute emergencies are eminently suitable for homoeopathic first-aid and self-help treatment. The following remedies are a valuable addition to any home medicine cabinet and indications for their use in emergencies are simple. Those marked with an asterisk are contained in the home remedy kit and full instructions for the use of each remedy are included. Unless otherwise indicated, they are supplied in the 30th potency.

ACONITUM NAPELLUS,* Aconite, monkshood. Principal indications: **SHOCK, FEVER** and the after-effects of **FRIGHT**

For shock, croup and the effects of frights or chills; any emergencies such as accidents, animal bites, asthma, haemorrhage, bereavement etc.; if there is fear, distress, breathlessness, palpitations, trembling or numbness and tingling. Use at the onset of fever if the patient is thirsty, restless or anxious, especially if the acute attack begins about 1 to 2 a.m.

ALLERGY REMEDIES. Principal indication: **ALLERGIES**

The remedies most commonly used are cat fur 30, dog hair 30, mixed grass pollens 30, horse dander 30 and house dust 200. They are invaluable where the patient is known to be allergic to these agents.

ALLIUM CEPA, Red onion. Principal indications: **COLDS** and **HAY FEVER**

A good remedy for an early cold or hay fever. There is sneezing with watery discharge from the nose which burns like fire and may excoriate the upper lip. The eyes may burn and smart and look red, but the discharge is bland. Lachrimation is worse indoors and in the evening and better outside, but the cough is worse in cold air. The inflammation soon spreads to the ears, nose and larynx.

ANTIMONIUM CRUDUM,* Black sulphide of antimony. Principal indication: STOMACH

For an upset stomach in a cross, touchy, depressed patient. For a baby who vomits feeds, has a white-coated tongue and cracks at the corners of the mouth. For lack of appetite and sick headaches from catarrh, alcohol or bathing. The patient wants sharp, sour drinks or pickles and is bloated with much belching.

ANTIMONIUM TARTARICUM,* Tartar emetic. Principal indication: COUGH with RATTLING CHEST

The patient is touchy, drowsy and very weak, cold with a clammy sweat, the face is pale or bluish and the tongue white-coated. There is breathlessness, suffocating, gasping for breath and the need to sit up. There is a rattling cough but an inability to cough up the phlegm. The patient is worse for warmth.

APIS MELLIFICA, Honey bee. Principal indications: INFLAMMATION with SWELLING and STINGING

Acute inflammation associated with swelling and redness, stinging and burning; with marked sensitivity of the affected part to any form of heat and relief from cold baths or bathing. Sore throats, hives, styes, insect bites, bee stings, allergic reactions with the above indications.

ARNICA,* Leopard's bane. Principal indications: INJURY and BRUISING

For bruises, sprains, concussion, crushed fingers, road accidents etc. If the patient is shocked give ACONITE first. Also for exhaustion and aching muscles from strain, sport or over-use. Use before and after dental surgery.

ARSENICUM ALBUM, ★ Arsenic trioxide. Principal indications: **VOMITING** and **DIARRHOEA**

For situations where sickness and diarrhoea occur simultaneously, for example, gastric flu, food poisoning and so on. The patient feels very cold and is anxious and *very* restless, exhausted but cannot rest. There are burning pains in the stomach, a thirst for small sips of warm drinks and a need for warmth. The patient cannot bear the sight or smell of food.

BELLADONNA, ★ Deadly nightshade. Principal indications: **EARACHE** and **FEVER**

For fever when the patient is burning hot, flushed, wide-eyed and excited, possibly delirious and cannot stand jarring noise or light. The patient must keep warm and is thirsty but will not drink. Belladonna is a specific for scarlet fever, which is rarely seen nowadays. It is used also for sore throats, colic, throbbing headaches, aching boils and severe earache with the above symptoms, and for the effects of sunstroke.

BRYONIA, ★ Wild hops. Principal indications: **PAIN** or **HEADACHES**

For bursting headaches, migraine, arthritis, pleurisy – especially if brought on by exposure to a cold east wind – and *only* if the pains are worse for movement, breathing or warmth, and better for pressure, lying still and keeping cool. The patient is grumpy, irritable, parched and thirsty for cold drinks.

CALENDULA OFFICINALIS, Marigold. Principal indication: **HEALING OF SORES**

A remarkable healing agent when applied locally, useful for open wounds and areas such as ulcers which will not heal. A haemostatic after tooth extraction. Use as the tincture or ointment.

CAMPHORA, ★ Camphor. Principal indication: **CHILL**

When icy cold following a chill. For the first stage of a cold or 'flu' when the patient is chilled, sneezing, better for warmth and feeling frozen. For diarrhoea brought on by chill.

CANTHARIS,* Spanish fly. Principal indications: **BLADDER INFECTIONS, CYSTITIS** and **BURNS**

For cystitis when the urine scalds and is passed drop by drop, associated with unbearable urgency and frequency. Also for burns and scalds which are better for cold applications and burning itchy blisters. For gnat and midge bites.

CARBO VEGETABILIS,* Vegetable charcoal. Principal indications: **WIND** and **COLLAPSE**

For use when the stomach is much distended, passing wind upwards and possibly down. The patient must sit up and loosen clothing. For collapse if the patient is pale or bluish, pulseless, cold, with cold sweat, needs propping up, gasping for breath, must have air and, although cold, likes to be fanned.

CHAMOMILLA,* Chamomile. Principal indications: **FRANTIC PAIN** and **TEETHING BABIES**

For unbearable pains, earache, toothache, teething, better for being picked up, one cheek red and hot, the other pale. Also for colic and diarrhoea with green motions in a bad-tempered, impatient patient, who is worse for heat and anger.

COLOCYNTHIS,* Bitter cucumber. Principal indication: **COLIC**

For agonizing colicky pain, better for doubling up, hard pressure, heat and twisting about. Very restless. Griping pains causing distension, belching and vomiting and sometimes diarrhoea. Colic and neuralgia from anger and 'getting worked up'. Dysmenorrhoea. All complaints often brought on by anger.

EUPHRASIA,* Eyebright. Principal indications: **MEASLES** and **HAY FEVER**

For the onset of measles when the eyes are streaming, the tears burn and the patient cannot stand light. Running nose, sneezing and cough, throbbing headache and hay fever with the above symptoms. Worse indoors, worse for warmth and worse in the evenings.

FERRUMPHOSPHORICUM, Iron phosphate. Principal indications: **COLDS** and **NOSE-BLEEDS**

For the first stage of inflammation such as early fevers, colds or other viral infections or earache when the patient is flushed and hot, often has red cheeks and is sensitive to cold and cold air (cf. BELLADONNA where the whole face is flushed). The FERRUM PHOSPHORICUM patient is more alert than the BELLADONNA patient and less fearful and anxious than the ACONITE patient. There may be a tendency to nose-bleeds and there is often a dry cough.

GELSEMIUM,* Yellow jasmine. Principal indications: **INFLUENZA** and **NERVOUS DEBILITY**

For use when the patient is feeling hot, flushed, aching, trembling, dizzy, drowsy and feeling 'drugged' or 'weak and wobbly'. There is headache, the limbs and eyes feel heavy, the back is chilly and there is sneezing, a running nose, sore throat and difficulty in swallowing. No thirst. It is used also for upsets from 'nerves'.

HEPAR SULPHURIS CALCAREUM, Hahnemann's calcium sulphide. Principal indications: **ABSCESSES, ULCERS** and **BOILS** in an **IRRITABLE** patient.

There is physical hypersensitivity and mental irritability. The patient is hypersensitive to touch, cold and pain and there is a tendency to suppuration. For the early stages of boils, ulcers, abscesses etc. There is often an offensive, sour sweat and smelly feet. Abscesses are better for local warmth.

HYPERCAL, a mixture of hypericum and calendula. Principal indication: **HEALING OF SORES**

The action is similar to that of calendula but is often much more effective. Used for the healing of wounds, sores, ulcers etc. Use as the tincture: 2 to 3 drops in 1 to 2 pints of water, or as the ointment.

HYPERICUM, St John's-wort. Principal indication: **NERVE INJURIES**

For nerve injuries associated with pain and for incised, lacerated or contused wounds when the pains are severe and possibly of long duration. Also for the consequences of spinal concussion.

IPECACUANHA,* Ipecac-root. Principal indications: **NAUSEA** and **COUGH**

For persistent nausea, possibly with vomiting, and a *clean* tongue and much saliva. For the onset of violent, suffocating wheezing bouts and coughing. Also for nose-bleeds and haemorrhages associated with nausea.

KALI BICHROMICUM, Potassium bichromate. Principal indications: **COUGH** with **THICK, STRINGY CATARRH** or **PHLEGM**

There are thick, stringy, gelatinous, or ropy green or yellow discharges fron the mucous membranes of the eyes, ears, nose or throat. Symptoms come and go suddenly and pains wander from place to place. Joint pains often alternate with diarrhoea, respiratory problems or digestive upsets. Such patients get cold easily and are worse in warm or hot weather. The cough is often worse at 2 to 3 a.m.

LACHESIS, the venom of the Bushmaster or Surukuku snake. Principal indications: **SORE THROATS, BOILS** and **ABSCESSES**

For sore throats, boils, abscesses and menstrual pain when the symptoms are more intense on waking from sleep, in a loquacious, jealous, suspicious and excitable patient. Symptoms are often worse on the left side of the body, or begin on the left side and move to the right. The patient is sensitive to the pressure of clothing, especially round the throat and waist. The eyes may be sensitive to light, noise irritates and light touch upsets, though firm pressure may be comforting. They often crave open air and prefer cool temperatures to heat though any extremes of temperature make them weak. Inflamed areas are usually dark blue or purplish.

LEDUM PALUSTRE, Marsh tea. Principal indication: **PUNCTURED** or **PENETRATING WOUNDS**

Useful for stings and puncture wounds, particularly wounds which are sensitive to touch, tender abscesses and septic conditions relieved by cold, and for splinters under the nail. The pains are worse for heat and better for cold. Also for injuries to the eye or around the eye and nose. Often follows **ARNICA** well.

MAGNESIA PHOSPHORICA, Magnesium phosphate. Principal indication: **COLICKY PAIN**

Useful in dysmenorrhoea (menstrual pain) where the pains double the patient up, are better for pressure and local heat and worse for cold. Also for flatulent colic associated with belching of wind which gives no relief. In children the legs may be drawn up. Also for neuralgia often with pain behind the right ear. The colics of **MAGNESIA PHOSPHORICA** are not precipitated by anger as they are in **COLOCYNTH**.

MERCURIUS SOLUBILIS,* Mercury. Principal indication: **FEVERISH COLD**

For use when the patient is feeling chilly in the cold and hot in warmth, weak and trembling with offensive sweat and breath. There is profuse greenish catarrh and much salivation, thirst and diarrhoea with persistent straining, passing slime and possibly also blood. All symptoms are worse at night.

NATRUM MURIATICUM,* Sodium chloride, common salt. Principal indications: **RECURRENT COLDS** and **DEPRESSION**

For 'sneezy' colds with cold sores and if there is much nasal catarrh; if the patient is feeling cold but worse in a warm room. The patient has a greasy skin, likes salt, is thirsty, irritable, weary and possibly weepy. Seek doctor's advice on depression. Do *not* attempt to self-treat.

NUX VOMICA,* Poison-nut. Principal indications: **STOMACH AILMENTS** and **FLU**

For a chilly, irritable and possibly quarrelsome patient with delayed indigestion, nausea, constipation or frequent, unsatisfactory bowel actions; itching piles; flu or raw throat, if chilled when uncovered. Stuffy colds and if the patient is worse in cold air; snuffles in irritable infants.

PHOSPHORUS.* Principal indication: **LARYNGITIS** and **REPEATED VOMITING**

For use when the chest is tight, the patient is hoarse and it hurts to talk; possibly there is loss of voice. Dry, tickling, racking cough, worse in cold air and worse talking. Gastritis with a craving for cold drinks which may be vomited immediately. Nervousness and thunder headaches.

PODOPHYLLUM, May-apple. Principal indication: **FLATULENT GASTRO-ENTERITIS**

Useful in children with symptoms of gastro-enteritis, colicky pains and bilious vomiting. The stool is gushing and offensive, often occurring early in the morning or during teething in a child with hot, glowing cheeks. Patient can lie comfortably only on the stomach. The abdomen is distended with much rumbling and gurgling of wind. Constipation may alternate with the diarrhoea and there is much flatus with the stool.

PULSATILLA,* Wind flower. Principal indications: **CATARRH** and **MEASLES**

For thick-coloured catarrh of the eyelids and nose, loss of smell and dry mouth with *no* thirst. The patient is better in the open air; catarrhal cough worsens in a warm room. Also for measles and indigestion from fat and rich food.

RHUS TOXICODENDRON,* Poison-ivy. Principal indications: **RHEUMATISM** and **ARTHRITIS**

For pain and stiffness which is worse in wet weather and cold air, in bed and after rest. Better for movement, though the first movements hurt. Better keeping moving. For flu and a dry cough with the above symptoms. Also for itching blisters and shingles if the patient is restless. Tendon sprains.

RUTA, Rue. Principal indications: **TENDON** and **LIGA-MENT SPRAINS** and **STRAINS**

Useful for synovial membranes and pain associated with peri-osteal injuries, bruises which leave indurations and hardened masses on tendons. Sciatica worse lying down at night, associated with the restlessness of RHUS TOXICODENDRON and the bruised sensation of ARNICA.

SPONGIA TOSTA, Roasted sponge. Principal indications: **CROUP** and **BARKING COUGH**

A good remedy for croup and dry, barking coughs with hoarse-ness, as if the larynx is dry, burning and constricted. Respiration may be difficult as in asthma. Symptoms abate after eating and drinking. The cough seems to come from a spot deep in the chest.

SULPHUR. * Principal indication: **SKIN RASHES**

For burning, itching skin rashes which are worse for warmth, scratching, washing and wearing clothes. Burning boils, styes and piles. The patient is hungry, tires easily, has hot 'flushes', morning diarrhoea and hot feet which are uncovered in bed.

SYMPHYTUM, Comfrey or knitbone. Principal indication: **FRACTURES**

For use in wounds affecting the bones and in the non-union of fractures, traumatic injuries to the eye and injuries to sinews, tendons and the periosteum. It appears to act on bone and joints generally.

URTICA URENS, Stinging nettle. Principal indication: **BURNS**

This will give almost instant relief of pain in burns and scalds with rapid healing. Even old burns that are not healing will res-pond. It is helpful used locally for bee stings and angioneurotic oedema. Use as the tincture, cream or ointment.

Appendix 2 Avoidance of Exposure to House-Dust Mite

BEDS AND BEDDING

This is the most important consideration. Pillows may be washable, non-allergic or Terylene. Mattresses should be of solid foam or a new upholstered mattress, covered before use with a good quality plastic or PVC cover. The cover prevents any penetration of skin scales or mites into the mattress, whether foam or upholstered, and has the advantage that it is easily wiped clean. It is the skin scales which provide the mites with their food source. Any new upholstered mattress is fully infested with house-dust mites within three months if it is not covered before use. Covering an already used mattress with a plastic or vinyl cover leads to the growth of moulds in the mattress and should only be done as a short-term measure – that is one to two months at the most. Acrilan or polyester underblankets are available to counteract the cold feel of the plastic cover and to prevent slipping of the overlying bed-clothes.

All sheets, blankets, quilts or duvets must be readily washable and should be thoroughly washed and aired every two to three months. Materials such as Polyester/cotton, Acrilan and Dacron are ideal. Using these materials, it is possible to wash the underblanket, blankets and duvets in the morning, and even in winter have them dried and back on the bed by evening. This saves having to duplicate blankets, quilts etc. in order to achieve the mandatory two-to-three-monthly wash.

The base of the bed should be of simple springs or wooden slats and not an upholstered divan base, unless covered with a good plastic or PVC cover.

OTHER POINTS TO WATCH

● Soft toys such as teddy bears and golliwogs can become infested with house-dust mites as readily as bedding. These should therefore be made of washable materials and treated similarly to the bed.

● Sufferers from house-dust-mite allergy should not sleep in, or bounce on, other beds unless they have been treated in a similar fashion to their own.

● If there is more than one bed in the patient's room, then these other beds must also be treated, otherwise there will be an 'aerosol' effect of house-dust mites from the beds with every movement of their occupants.

● Children must be advised not to bounce on upholstered furniture, crawl under beds or hide in wardrobes.

● Vacuuming of carpets must not be done in the presence of house-dust sufferers and preferably not within two hours of their being around.

● If the sufferer is a housewife, it is advisable that all the beds in the house be treated so that she does not become exposed when dealing with the beds of other members of the family. She should also either get someone else to do the vacuuming for her or else wear an efficient mask while performing this task.

● Ducted-air central heating must be avoided since this spreads house-dust mites throughout the whole atmosphere of the house.

HOLIDAYS

The problem of sleeping arrangements while on holiday is easily dealt with. Patients should take their own pillow, a large sheet of good quality plastic and a washable sleeping-bag (and blankets if desired). The plastic is spread over the entire bed and the sleeping-bag and pillow are placed on top. Ideally there should be no one else sharing the room.

Appendix 3 Useful Addresses

The Faculty of Homoeopathy
Royal London Homoeopathic Hospital
Great Ormond Street
LONDON WCIN 3HR

The British Homoeopathic Association
27a Devonshire Street
LONDON WIN IRJ

The Homoeopathic Development Foundation Limited
19a Cavendish Square
LONDON WIM 9AD

The Hahnemann Society
Humane Education Centre
Avenue Lodge
Bounds Green Road
LONDON N22 4EU

The National Association of Homoeopathic Groups
Easter Cottage
School Lane
Middleton Stoney
OXON

A. Nelson and Company Limited
For counter sales:
  Nelson Pharmacies
  73 Duke Street
  Grosvenor Square
  LONDON WIM 6BY

For postal requests:
  A. Nelson and Company
  5 Endeavour Way
  Wimbledon
  LONDON SWI9 9UH

For home remedy kits:
    Freeman's Pharmaceuticals and Homoeopathic Chemists
    7 Eaglesham Road
    Clarkston
    GLASGOW G76 7BU

    Ainsworths Homoeopathic Pharmacy
    38 New Cavendish Street
    LONDON WIM 7LH

    The Bristol Homoeopathic Hospital
    Cotham Road
    BRISTOL BS6 6JU

    The Glasgow Homoeopathic Hospital
    1000 Great Western Road
    GLASGOW G12 0NR

    The Liverpool Homoeopathic Clinic
    The Department of Homoeopathic Medicine
    The Mossley Hill Hospital
    Park Road
    LIVERPOOL L18

    The Manchester Homoeopathic Clinic
    Brunswick Street
    MANCHESTER M13 9ST

    The Royal London Homoeopathic Hospital
    Great Ormond Street
    LONDON WCIN 3HR

    The Tunbridge Wells Homoeopathic Hospital
    Church Road
    Tunbridge Wells
    KENT

Appendix 4 Suggestions for Further Reading

Boyd, Hamish, *Introduction to Homoeopathic Medicine*, Beaconsfield Publishers Limited, 1981.

Blackie, Margery G., *The Patient, Not the Cure*, Macdonald and Jane's, 1976.

Clover, Anne, *Homoeopathy: A Patient's Guide*, Thorsons Publishers Limited, Wellingborough, 1984.

Homoeopathy for the Family, 3rd edition, the Homocopathic Development Foundation Limited, 1983.

Karagulla, Shafica, *Breakthrough to Creativity*, De Vorss & Co., Santa Monica, Calif., 1974.

MacLeod, George, *Homoeopathy for Pets*, 2nd edition, the Homoeopathic Development Foundation Limited, 1983.

Pert, J. C., *The Family Prescriber*, Wigmore Publications Limited, 1984.

Gibson, Sheila L. M., Templeton, Louise and Gibson, Robin G., *Cook Yourself a Favour: 350 Recipes to Help you Help Yourself to Better Health*, 2nd edition, Thorsons Publishers Limited, Wellingborough, 1986.

Jones, Frank Pierce, *Body Awareness in Action*, Schocken Books, New York, 1976.

Alexander, F. Matthias, *The Use of the Self*, Re-educational Publications Limited, 1946.

Milner, Dennis and Smart, Edward, *The Loom of Creation*, Neville Spearman, 1975.

Burr, Harold Saxton, *Blueprint for Immortality: The Electrical Patterns of Life*, Neville Spearman, 1972.

INDEX